EXTRAORDINARY HEALING STORIES

Michel-Charles SULTAN

ABOUT THE AUTHOR

Born on May 23, 1959, in Constantine, Michel-Charles SULTAN is a licensed physiotherapist who earned his diploma in Paris in 1984.

In 1987, he joined the Antares Association and trained under Mr. Eddie COPPRY in kinesiology, specifically "Touch for Health," a method developed by American chiropractors Drs. Goodheart, Bennett, and Chapman.

He continued his studies in Switzerland, earning a diploma in osteopathy from the Geneva College of Osteopathy in 1997.

A practitioner of Traditional Chinese Medicine (TCM), he trained for three years in Brussels, Belgium, at the Europe-Shanghai College under the guidance of Francis LENDERS, obtaining his diploma in 2002.

Throughout his 40-year professional career, he has relentlessly explored and questioned the body as the unconscious keeper of life's trials. These daily wounds are stored at the heart of our cells: our cellular memory.

His dual somatic and emotional approach provides each of us the opportunity to become aware of the subtle, invisible connections that punctuate and shape our biological responses. This constant adaptation to the external world emerges as a survival strategy, perfectly mirroring emotionally unmanageable situations experienced and felt as dramatic, often in isolation.

His investigative work unfolds like a personal, familial, and transgenerational inquiry, particularly following his discovery in 2004 of psycho-genealogy tools.

Moreover, he had the privilege of working as a physiotherapist-osteopath in two psychiatric clinics in Île-de-France during the second half of his career, spanning nearly 20 years.

Today, he gives conferences to promote and share with as many people as possible this revolutionary approach that lies at the crossroads of disciplines.

DISCLAIMER TO THE READER

This book cannot, under any circumstances, be considered a medical method, a treatment technique, or a discovery.

This approach strictly requires and relies on medical diagnoses, adherence to medical treatments, and protocols in accordance with current scientific and medical knowledge.

Any person refusing to seek medical care for themselves or others assumes full and sole responsibility for their decision.

It is important to emphasize, in the interest of honesty with the reader, that this book, intended for the general public, is the result of many years of consultations. It is thanks to the shared and reciprocal trust of patients that the path of this therapeutic evolution began.

I would like to specify here that this approach is the outcome of a journey gradually enriched over the years by accumulated experiences, seminars, and teachings from my professors and mentors.

May they all be thanked here for passing on the fruits of their knowledge and expertise.

This learning process encompasses multiple facets, each reflecting a spark of truth. This slow construction has been marked by successes, which have fueled my passion for caregiving and my quest for a more comprehensive, holistic, and intimate understanding.

Equally, numerous challenges have allowed me to grow with the certainty that absolute truth does not exist and that it contains different realities unique to each individual.

This therapeutic tool is the result of a synthesis based on:

- A mechanistic approach: physiotherapy and osteopathy,

- An energetic approach: kinesiology and Traditional Chinese Medicine,

- A neurolinguistic approach: conversational hypnosis and neurolinguistic programming (NLP),

- A biopsychological approach: total biology of living beings and biological codes of diseases,

- A transgenerational approach: analysis of family history and intergenerational transmissions.

For clarity, I emphasize that I am not the inventor of any method. The results of this approach, as well as its merit, belong entirely to the mentors who trained me.

My sincere thanks go to all the contributors to this wonderful journey and to all the ordinary heroes of these extraordinary stories.

INTRODUCTION

In recent years, we have witnessed a revolution in our understanding and approach to diseases. The third millennium is beginning with a new perspective. Indeed, several authors have established a connection between emotional experiences and the somatization of illnesses. Groundbreaking research is reshaping and illuminating the relationship between the psyche and organic diseases, providing the general public with a unique way to understand the invisible links between the emotions that punctuate our lives and our biological responses.

The internet and social networks now act as vehicles, connecting 21st-century individuals to this new body of knowledge, which is accessible to everyone. Questioning one's illness—why it appears, its location, its timing, its progression, and its cycles—has become a crucial step in the healing process in light of these advancements. This broader perspective of the human being, faced with the challenges of illness, offers answers to deeper and more meaningful questions:

- Finding meaning in this struggle, this battle.

- Understanding that this challenge is neither a curse nor a matter of fate dictated by chance.

- Exercising free will with full awareness of the available therapies and treatments.

- Recognizing that decoding the unconscious program behind the illness is a crucial step in personal evolution, providing everyone the opportunity to share the fruits of these new approaches with humanity.

This immense work of synthesis and analysis has established a fundamental link between feelings, emotional experiences, and biological responses. These responses, inscribed in our tissues, represent the brain's optimal solution to ensure and prolong our survival in a hostile environment where surrounding dangers trigger stress.

Understanding these survival archetypes allows us, through awareness, to better manage our health and restore both physical and mental well-being. To clarify, this body of work demonstrates a direct reality: our emotions are deeply connected to our illnesses. It is essential to specify that the term EMOTION here refers to intense, destabilizing, and life-altering psychological shocks.

These events are emotional TSUNAMIS, leaving the individual in a state of shock, without a strategy for response, mental adaptation, or defense—a true state of stupor.

This feeling is imprinted deep in our tissues, organs, and cells, programming a disease or behavioral disorder. Indeed, to ensure survival, the brain uses the organ and its function to provide a bodily solution when the mind cannot find one. The cost, of course, is the illness, but the individual is kept alive, as mental stress decreases once the body takes over.

It is crucial to understand that prolonged mental stress or shock has the power to lead to death. Intense stress periods eliminate the focus necessary for survival, while the lack of rest leads to physical exhaustion. Mental function begins to recover, almost normally, once biological adaptation is in place. Through this transfer from brain to body, the individual gains time...

It is this time that must be used to reverse the morbid process, freeing the body, which is the instrument trapped by our emotions. It is possible to resolve the mental conflict that triggered the illness and thus free the body from its temporary adaptation mission.

The therapeutic approach proposed here rests on two essential pillars:

1. **A precise medical diagnosis,** established through complementary examinations to identify as rigorously as possible:

- The tissues,
- The organs,
- The joints,
- The systems... where the illness resides.

2. **Simultaneously initiating a psycho-emotional approach,** recognizing that the body is not just a machine or instrument but also the receptacle of our emotions. If these emotions are not verbalized or brought to consciousness, they crystallize in our bodies, but not just anywhere—they resonate precisely with our life history.

Listening to one's illness means accepting to hear what the "dis-ease" is saying in your body.

- "What is expressed is not imprinted and fades away."

- "What is not expressed is imprinted in your body."

To illustrate this knowledge, we invite readers to join us in exploring extraordinary genealogical stories from everyday life.

THESE EXTRAORDINARY STORIES WANDER… FROM GENERATION TO GENERATION.

Let us rediscover our family tree and roots. Let us travel into and explore our genealogical universe…

LET US LISTEN CONSCIOUSLY TO THIS GENIUS LOGIC.

Story No. 1:

WATER ALLERGY OR THE MEMORY OF A FAMILY TRAGEDY

This story takes place in Côte d'Ivoire, in Abidjan, West Africa, on the Atlantic coast, over forty years ago. Today, our patient resides in France, where he consults in Paris, desperately seeking a cure for a water allergy that causes him many daily troubles. In succession, a general practitioner, a dermatologist, and finally an allergist all confirm, backed by allergy tests, the diagnosis of a water allergy. Medical treatments are implemented and accompanied by all the usual precautions for body care:

- Soothing and hypoallergenic creams and ointments,
- Topical cortisone,
- Oral antihistamines,
- Repairing sprays and body lotions,
- The use of appropriate laundry detergents and soaps.

The patient suffers from itching, swelling, and red patches covering large areas of his body, with very few areas spared. His daily life quickly turns into a nightmare: he no longer dares to wash or take a shower. A simple bath soon becomes hell. Of course, he avoids contact with the irritant, but this does not resolve his skin problem, which flares up with each exposure. His fear grows with each medical consultation, along with his stress and confusion. He desperately seeks a solution.

In our society, we are witnessing a significant increase in allergies linked to changes in our lifestyles. Most of these allergies are related to food, respiratory issues, medications, or insect venom. However, medical professionals assert that patients' allergic reactions to water are not caused by water molecules but by substances contained within the water: minerals, organic compounds, microorganisms, and even the temperature of cold water. This uncommon condition is referred to as hydro-allergies, the true causes of which remain largely unexplained, with their mechanisms evading medical science's understanding.

However, none of these hypotheses offer a solution for our patient. In light of this therapeutic failure, Bernard, following his allergist's advice, agrees to pursue a psycho-emotional approach.

Investigation:

This involves compiling a file detailing all the important events in our patients' life histories.

- Name: Mr. A. Bernard
- Date of Birth: 01/19/1970
- Place of Birth: Abidjan, Côte d'Ivoire
- Profession: Computer Scientist
- Eldest of two boys: Bernard and Alain, born 08/07/1975 in Abidjan

Reason for consultation:

Contact allergy to water (it is worth noting here that our patient can drink water without any issues).

Questions :

- How does one develop an allergy to water, an essential and indispensable substance for life?
- How and in what way does this symptom or illness reveal a dramatic part of this family's history?

History:

Before the tragedy, on a beautiful sunny morning in July 1979, Albertine, accompanied by her two boys, Bernard and Alain, went to Abidjan's covered market. On the way, she decided to let the two children sunbathe on the beach. She entrusted the supervision of Alain to his older brother Bernard, strictly forbidding any swimming in her absence. The rules were clear. Upon her return, a real tragedy unfolded. She found the lifeless body of her youngest child, despite the rescuers' efforts to bring him back to life. Unable to contain her emotion, she screamed accusatory words that would forever be etched in Bernard's memory: "You carry the death of your little brother; you are responsible, and he died because of you."

Reflections:

The body does not create a symptom or illness without meaning.

This response is always orchestrated, intelligent, and echoes a stress, an unmanageable situation, or an unresolved issue experienced by a member of the family or one of their ancestors or descendants.

How is this somatic response a solution for the family? How is it beneficial?

In this approach, it is essential to allow the patient to access the scenario of the tragedy, the emotions that the automatic brain carefully recorded in the unconscious to spare the conscious mind from constantly reliving unbearable mental suffering. During the therapeutic session, it is crucial to identify the moment of shock so that the person can connect with the episode related to the stress. Therefore, we provide the patient with a spatial and temporal frame of reference, allowing them to reconnect with the information stored in their memory. I ask Bernard directly, "When did water become dangerous or represent a threat in your life?" His immediate response: "The drowning of my four-year-old brother Alain."

At that moment, Bernard understands the previously invisible connection between this tragedy and his allergic response, with water being the emotional trigger of this tragic event.

GENO-SOCIOGRAM

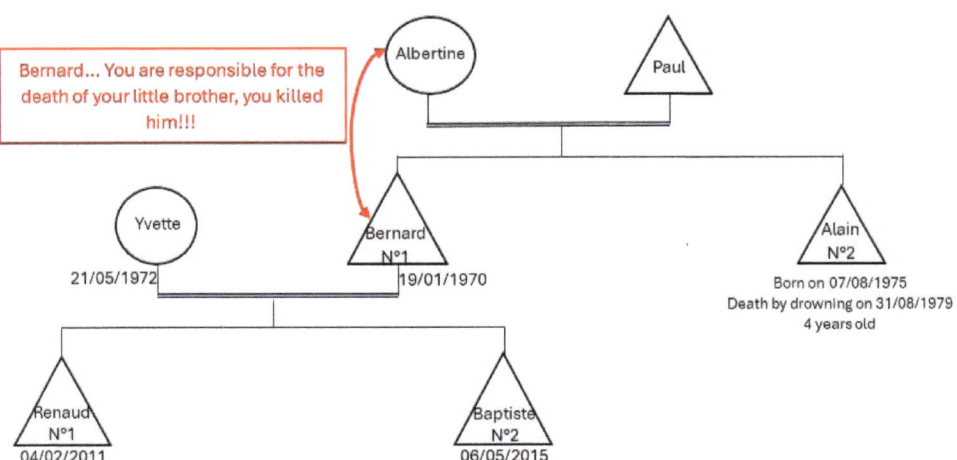

He then inquires about how to heal: by simply recognizing and accepting the connection. This awareness is crucial for healing and the reversible process of pathologies. However, he shares his doubts due to feelings of responsibility and guilt. While his reaction is completely understandable, it is the therapist's job to reframe the situation and remind the patient of these key points:

• A nine-year-old child cannot be responsible for supervising a four-year-old.

• His attention and awareness of danger were not fully developed; he was too young to bear this responsibility, and his focus was easily distracted.

• Even adults cannot maintain constant supervision for 100% of the time and space: an impossible task.

• The safety of these two children should have been entrusted to an adult.

Only then does he accept to let go of this weight of guilt and responsibility. His brain integrates the explanations, but he still does not understand why: "If the tragedy happened forty years ago, why did my water allergy only manifest so late in my life?"

Letting go and mourning:

The brain continuously revisits and connects anniversary dates when symptoms appear or reappear. I explain to Bernard that the triggering factor for his allergy arose when his eldest son, Renaud, celebrated his ninth birthday—the same age when the tragedy of his younger brother's death occurred. This unconscious emotional stress triggered the allergic symptom, allowing Bernard to express, through his biology, a conflict imprinted in his unconscious mind, thus enabling him to finally mourn this tragedy. The symptom gains clarity, providing him insight into its deeper meaning. The message is communicated to the family: heightened vigilance and attention for Baptiste, the second child, reminiscent of Alain, who was also the second child.

Since that single consultation, Bernard's symptoms have completely vanished, leaving no trace... No recurrence to date, allowing him to return to his normal life.

Story No. 2:

OBSESSIVE-COMPULSIVE DISORDER: KNOCK KNOCK, WHO'S THERE?

Catherine made an appointment at my osteopathy clinic for a routine case of lower back pain located at the third lumbar vertebra (L3). During the consultation, she described the circumstances surrounding the onset of the symptom: lumbar pain following the lifting of heavy loads and housework. I then proceeded with the usual mechanical tests:

- Palpation tests,
- Mobility tests,
- Resistance tests,
- Checking for painful points, trigger points, and alarm points.

Consultation No. 1:

Medical History:

- No significant medical history,
- Normal digestive tests: the patient has a good appetite and regular bowel movements,
- Normal radiological tests: no mechanical or chronic fragility like arthritis, osteoporosis, decalcification, or spondylolisthesis,
- Normal biological tests (blood, liver, kidney function),
- Neurological history: she has been followed for five years for **OCD** (**O**bsessive-**C**ompulsive **D**isorder).

As she explained her condition, Catherine immediately reached into her bag to show me the medication she couldn't find:

"I'm sorry, I must have left it on the kitchen table. By the way," she said, sitting up in her chair, "do you know what OCD is?"

I replied:

"Yes, but I prefer that you describe it to me because I have no opinion or expertise on the prescription of this neuroleptic."

She confirmed that she has been diligently following the treatment prescribed by her neurologist for five consecutive years, without significant results in her daily life. She then told me the following story:

At the age of 20, she was hired as a secretary-accountant in a family-run construction company. She held this position for about 17 years in a large office shared with five or six colleagues. At the age of 37, she was dismissed following a decision by occupational health, being declared "disabled" and unfit for her position. Since then, she has received an allowance from the COTOREP (Commission for the Orientation and Professional Reclassification of the Disabled), now the MDPH (Departmental House for Disabled Persons). She is now 41 years old. The loss of income forced her to move back in with her parents nearly five years ago.

She also undergoes psychotherapy once a week to help manage the stress resulting from the loss of her job, income, and autonomy.

While completing her file, I tried to understand her **<u>OCD</u>**:

She gets up several times a day, 15 to 20 times, to obsessively check the window handles, repeatedly testing the "open-close" mechanism. It's stronger than her, irrepressible, uncontrollable. Her colleagues became concerned and reported her behavior to their superiors, worried for her health and this troubling behavior.

Reflections:

If we accept that this response is tied to her personal history, linked to a survival-related stress or that of a family member, then this OCD is neither incoherent nor anarchic but perfectly orchestrated by the unconscious brain. This disorder must be viewed as a symptom of a deeper suffering buried in her life story.

Questions:

- What purpose does this OCD serve?
- In what way is it a solution, given that it caused her to lose her job, income, and autonomy?

I then asked her:

"Ms. Catherine, what is the purpose of a window, please?"

Surprised, she responded with a tight smile:

"To look through, to see outside."

"What else, please?"

"To ventilate a room, to get fresh air."

"What else, please?" I insisted.

She hesitated:

"I just answered you!"

I persisted:

"What else, please?"

Then, to stress her further, I added:

"This is a simple question for a child in elementary school."

She didn't understand my insistence or the purpose of my question. Her stress increased, and her brain searched desperately for an answer but couldn't articulate it. She couldn't recall the conflicting situation that triggered her OCD. A heavy silence settled for a few seconds, which seemed like an eternity.

I then clearly said the following:

"Constantly checking the windows... serves to prevent someone from coming in or going out."

At that exact moment, she accessed the long-buried situation. Her shoulders slumped, she curled up in her chair, her neck sank into her shoulders, her eyes lowered, and she burst into tears. Her face turned crimson, tears streaming down her flushed cheeks as her entire body shook with spasms. Gasping for breath, she struggled to find air. At that moment, I heard the cries of a 12- or 13-year-old child. It was no longer an adult sitting in front of me. After a few minutes, I said to her:

"While you close your eyes and cry in front of me, your unconscious brain is reconstructing an image, a vision, a scene, a sequence."

She nodded affirmatively.

"Can you talk about it?"

"Yes, we're at my parents' house, my little sister is nine years old, and I'm about to turn 13. We live in a single-story house in Champigny-sur-Marne (94), and we share the same bedroom. In the evening, our parents would come to kiss us goodnight, making sure to close the shutters, windows, and draw the curtains: 'Good night, children, sleep well, have sweet dreams.'

In the middle of the night, while Catherine was awake, the room was cold, the window wide open, and her little sister was no longer in her bed: she had run away through the window.

"What should I do?" she thought.

She decided not to close the window or the shutters, leaving the possibility for her sister to return. Her brain was stuck in an impasse.

Observations:

Closing the windows at night was a daily ritual shared between the parents and the children to ensure their safety.

Opening the window, however, was a solitary action taken to ensure her little sister's potential return.

These two actions—closing and opening—are contradictory and opposing. However, both actions ensured the safety of the two sisters: preventing an escape (closing) and allowing a return (opening). Therefore, checking the window handles became essential, hence the development of her OCD.

By mutual agreement, we postponed the osteopathy session for two weeks, allowing her brain enough time to enter a repair phase and dissolve the OCD. This realization helped Catherine grasp the invisible link between her sister's runaways and the onset of her OCD. I never asked Catherine why her sister had run away.

Epilogue:

Fifteen days later, Catherine returned for her second appointment, announcing that her OCD had improved by 80%. She no longer had to constantly check the window handles. Over time, she gradually reduced her medication and decided to retrain as an ATSEM (Specialized Territorial Agent for Nursery Schools). She found full-time employment, giving up her disability benefits. She moved into a new apartment near her parents and adopted a small dog for companionship. To this day, she has remained single and childless. I continued to see her for maintenance osteopathy sessions over many years without any recurrence of her OCD. Her sister got married and is now the mother of two little girls.

Story No. 3:

VAGINAL YEAST INFECTION OR THE ODYSSEY OF LIFE

This is the story of a 29-year-old woman who suffers from a vaginal yeast infection resistant to all conventional treatments, including recurring prescriptions of broad-spectrum antibiotics, pain relievers, and soothing creams.

Yeast infections, or vaginal candidiasis, cause itching and inflammation of the vulva and vaginal area. The cause is often attributed to yeasts, specifically *Candida albicans*. Her gynecologist, who has been treating her for over a year, explains that this condition is common after pregnancy due to a weakened immune system (from fatigue or breastfeeding), the use of oral contraceptives, or frequent vaginal douching. The doctor also mentions other possible factors, such as wearing synthetic clothing or exposure to inadequately disinfected pools, saunas, or hot tubs that promote the transmission of vaginal infections.

Rachel gave birth to her first child, a healthy boy named Samuel, weighing 3.52 kg, just a year ago. Both mother and child are doing well, except for this yeast infection that seems invincible despite the protocol put in place by her experienced 56-year-old obstetrician, a passionate doctor who is very attentive to his patients.

Naturally, he performed the necessary tests to identify the offending pathogen responsible for:

- Itching,

- Thick, foul-smelling discharge,

- White or yellowish discharge.

Besides these unpleasant symptoms, her intimacy with her partner has been disrupted, causing itching, burning, and skin irritation for him during intercourse. This has led the couple to use condoms as a preventive measure.

Despite following the treatment and hygiene measures rigorously, there has been no significant improvement. The condition persisted for seven years, alternating between periods of remission and recurrence. The calm periods were mostly observed during the breastfeeding phases of her next two pregnancies, as if the hormonal context related to life transmission muted the expression of the disease.

The worsening or remission of symptoms seemed to escape all medical logic.

The couple turned to alternative solutions, consulting naturopaths, dietitians, and aromatherapists, who recommended stricter dietary rules to strengthen the immune system while preserving intestinal health as much as possible.

Rachel was prescribed vaginal suppositories made from a blend of essential oils, based on an aromatogram—a test that determines the sensitivity or resistance of different germs (bacteria, viruses, mycobacteria) to essential oils. The term «aromatogram» was introduced by Dr. JEAN VALNET and Dr. MAURICE GIRAULT, the first clinicians in 1971 to test the germicidal power of aromatic oils and essences for treating diseases[1].

Despite the consultations and prescriptions, there was no significant improvement in her symptoms, and the couple remained in the same therapeutic impasse.

Rachel, wanting to protect her relationship and intimacy, searched the internet for solutions and testimonies about her health issue. One day, she stumbled upon information regarding a completely different approach to understanding and addressing her symptoms.

The Discovery

This new approach analyzed the conscious and unconscious emotional stresses experienced personally in one's life or resonated from the stresses of family members (ancestors or collateral relatives).

Rachel discovered that each of us can unconsciously harbor the unspoken secrets and silences of our family, an emotional and transgenerational inheritance.

Her readings and research led her to a deep conviction: she needed to understand what had happened in her family even before her conception and birth.

She decided to book an appointment with a therapist trained in psycho-genealogy.

During our session, I suggested constructing her geno-sociogram. This term, coined by Anne Ancelin Schützenberger

---

[1] Internet sources Wikipedia 04-2023

in her book *Psychogenealogy: Healing Family Wounds*[2], refers to a kind of family tree representing two, three, or four generations. This tree symbolizes and summarizes the relationships and information connecting the various family members, as well as the biomedical and psychosocial data related to them.

Excerpt from *Aïe, mes aïeux!* by Anne Ancelin Schützenberger:

"What matters is how the therapist perceives the individuals, the bonds that unite ancestors with their descendants and collateral relatives. These connections tell the invisible story of the clan through unspoken words, silences, gaps, and memory lapses that reveal much about what has been erased or struck from the family memory."

The geno-sociogram is the primary tool used to highlight patterns of repetition, accidents, illnesses, unresolved grief, anniversaries, and more.

This genealogical investigation relies on all official documents (records, birth, marriage, and death certificates, hospitalizations) and traces all significant events in the family's history (education, professions, divorces, separations, natural disasters, accidents, illnesses), as well as the emotional ties between all members of the family clan.

Here is Rachel's family tree. It contains relevant information about the members of her clan.

---

[2] Payot 2012

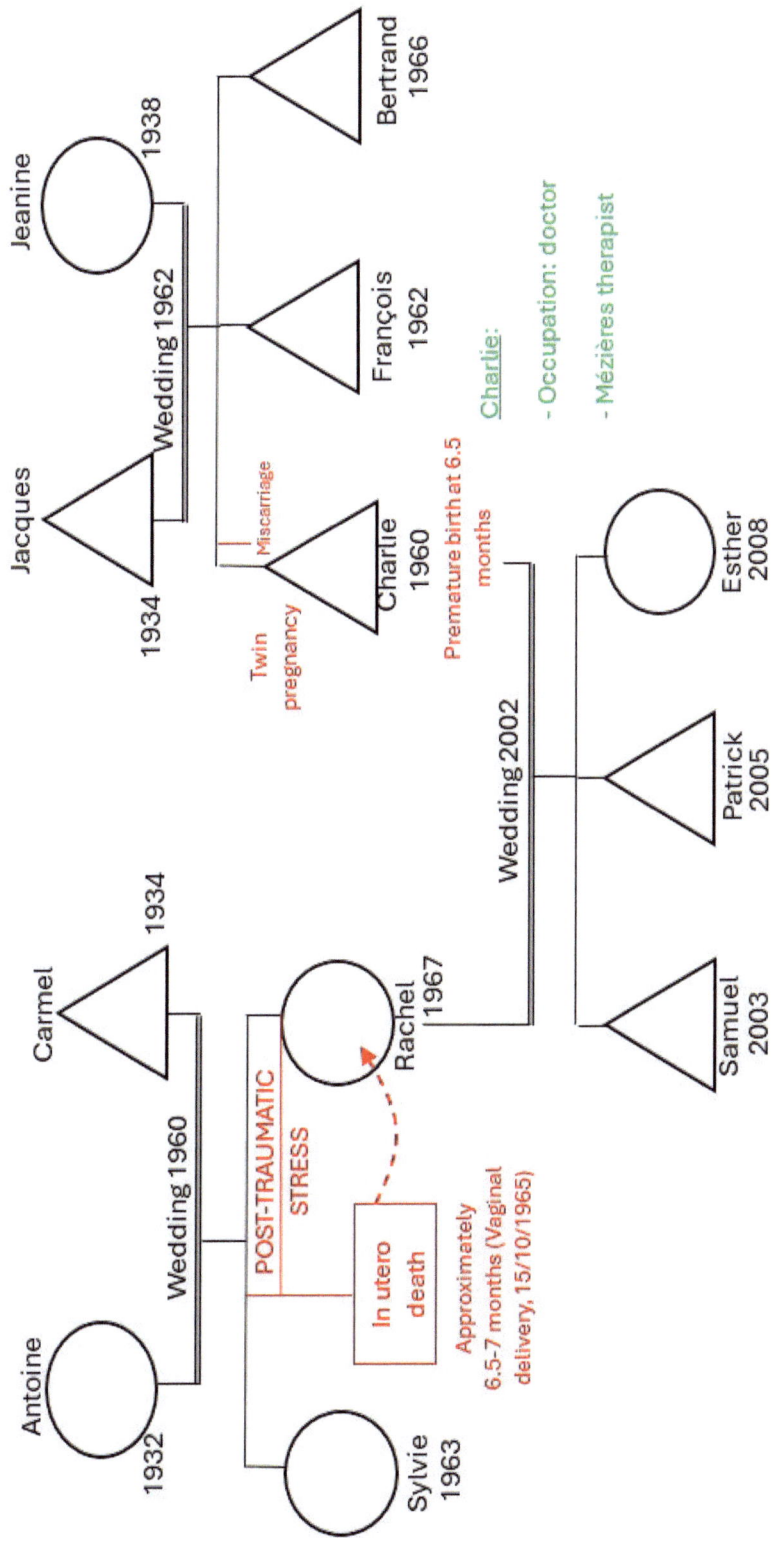

Consultation No. 1:

Upon reviewing her family tree, Rachel realized that while the family was intellectually aware of certain events, the invisible transmissions revealing the tragedies lived by her ancestors were less known.

Rachel was conceived after the tragedy of losing a 6.5 to 7-month-old baby, who died in utero in her mother Carmela's womb. The birth was still delivered vaginally.

Since the fetus was no longer driving its own birth, the obstetrician had to extract the stillborn baby, partially breaking the baby's skeleton during the process due to its rigidity. This procedure was carried out naturally without anesthesia or cesarean. Carmela felt, through all her senses and her entire body, each step of this forced delivery.

She recorded all the tactile, kinesthetic, auditory, olfactory, and visual stresses that accompanied this sad event.

This unavoidable and necessary step was carried out with the doctor's expertise, but it remained forever engraved in Carmela's emotional memory, known as «cellular memory» in genealogical terms.

Carmela had to go through the stages of grief: sadness, anger, confusion, and acceptance. Time passed, life went on, and little Rachel was born two years after this tragic episode.

Unknowingly, Rachel became the bearer of this memory. Throughout Carmela's third pregnancy, she lived in fear of reliving the same emotional pain, dreading a tragic outcome. Rachel, therefore, unconsciously absorbed all the stress her mother experienced and recorded:

- Before her conception, during the grieving process,

- During her time in utero, with maximum intensity between 6.5 to 7 months of gestation,

- At her birth, until her first cry, her first breath.

These emotions were unconsciously engraved in Rachel's brain and memory.

The rails of this tragedy were laid in Rachel's life path, and she was unconsciously tasked with finding a solution for her family's survival in this context.

Consultation No. 2:

The Meaning of the Symptom—Understanding the Ordeal

When a condition resists conventional treatment despite the care of medical professionals and the power of pharmacology, it is crucial to question the moral dimension related to life's sufferings and wounds.

This soul wound finds its expression in the symptom or illness etched in the patient's tissues.

WHAT DOES THIS VAGINAL YEAST INFECTION TELL US?

All major traditions cradle and nourish our collective unconscious. Nothing in the world is more sacred than the transmission of life, ensuring the survival of species and all life forms on Earth.

In this case, LIFE is no more, and the specter of DEATH taints the path of life.

In sacred texts, death is associated with impurity. Contact with corpses or dead bodies requires rituals of purification, prayers, or even periods of isolation symbolizing a cleansing process before returning to LIFE.

In nature, this role is assigned to fungi, bacteria, mycobacteria, and microorganisms responsible for decomposition, returning matter to the earth.

This yeast infection, on a cellular level, acts as a cleansing process for this impurity. It resonates with the fear of losing offspring and reactivates automatically during the conception of Rachel's first child, reawakening her mother's pain and sadness.

Consultation No. 3:

Healing the Family Tree with Awareness

In constructing a family tree, every detail, often the most insignificant, holds a part of the potential for healing.

This transgenerational approach teaches us that all children are the guardians and transmitters of unresolved emotional situations from their parents or ancestors. In other words, the parents' psychological conflict becomes the biological or behavioral manifestation in the child.

The illness expressed is always the optimal biological solution, perfectly responding to the psychological conflict experienced by the parents, ancestors, or sometimes even descendants.

The individual expresses, by proxy, illnesses that do not belong to them.

The brain never makes mistakes—it is programmed for survival, crafting the best solutions for the family members.

Questions & Answers

<u>How can Rachel repair her mother's moral pain?</u>

• When she becomes aware of the invisible links connecting her to her mother Carmela's moral pain, Rachel allows her brain to automatically activate the psychobiological repair program. The yeast infection is triggered to cleanse the impurity experienced by her mother.

• Rachel symbolically brings her mother a healthy 6.5-month-old premature baby by marrying Charlie, who was born prematurely and survived.

• Charlie, through his profession, helps heal the broken skeleton stress of the stillborn fetus. He is a Mézièriste and vertebrologist, treating and repairing the musculoskeletal system.

With this new psycho-genealogical understanding, Rachel realized that this new perspective shed light on her symptoms, offering a more holistic reading of her condition.

Within fifteen days of this transformative consultation, Rachel's vaginal tissue and mucosa began to heal.

Her symptoms have disappeared since 2003, with no recurrence following her conscious understanding. This emotional brain-based restitution enabled a full and complete healing.

This result was achieved through a new way of analyzing the symptom and its connection to the unconscious parental programs.

Understanding the various facets of this dramatic story allowed for the completion of the grieving process and the release of the unconscious conflict at the root of the physical issue.

Note on the Mézières Method

Developed by Françoise Mézières in 1947, this method of rehabilitation combines postures, massages, and stretches with breathing exercises to correct spinal deviations. The approach is based on correcting muscle chains to release neuromuscular tension. This work is rhythmically aligned with deep diaphragm breathing, with muscle tension release leading to spinal alignment. This technique is applied in the treatment of spinal conditions such as scoliosis, kyphosis, and kyphoscoliosis.

Story No. 4:

THE SOCIAL ELEVATOR OR THE FALL INTO VERTICALITY

This is the story of a woman around 60 years old who booked an appointment following a common case of lower back pain.

The date is November 4, 2012.

As I searched for Mrs. Françoise L.'s file in the computer to create a new session, I asked her to specify the reason for her visit: an accidental fall from standing height, caused by inattention, as she was hurrying through her daily tasks. While reviewing her past treatments from previous years, I was surprised to notice that Françoise had consulted me on the same date: between October 31 and November 5, in 2009, 2010, 2011, and now 2012...

Everything pointed to an accidental fall!

But how could mere chance orchestrate such a repetition?

Questions:

- Why does this happen at the same time every year?
- What significance does this period hold in her life story?
- Why the same week out of 52 weeks?

I was personally surprised by this calendar repetition. I asked her if this coincidence meant anything to her. Did this event, like an anniversary, evoke something in her memory?

"No," she replied.

She was unable to make a connection between these accidental falls and a specific memory related to her life.

I then asked her the following question:

"What is the biggest shock you experienced between October 31 and November 5, either recently or a long time ago, perhaps even very long ago?"

Immediately, her emotional, automatic, and unconscious brain did a quick review, and her response became clear:

"That date corresponds to the official date of my divorce."

History:

Françoise and Robert had been married for 35 years. They had three children and were the heads of a thriving SME with no fewer than 300 employees—a small gem they had built through their hard work in the microcomputing industry. For 30 years, Françoise had been a devoted executive assistant, working alongside her husband while also being a nurturing mother to their three children, providing love and affection within the home.

Their success was truly the result of a partnership between her and her husband, who held the position of CEO. Even though she worked in her husband's shadow, she organized, planned, and orchestrated all the necessary meetings for the company's growth.

As they approached retirement, Françoise expected to enjoy her time with her husband, surrounded by their children and grandchildren, finally enjoying well-deserved rest. Together, they had seemingly climbed every step of the social ladder. They lived in a grand mansion in the Yvelines (78), complete with a limousine, chauffeur, housekeeper, gardener, and cook. The house was nestled in a magnificent park with a pond, woods, and century-old trees.

But fate had other plans.

Robert hired a young executive assistant who, over time, replaced Françoise in decision-making roles at the company. Eventually, Robert asked Françoise for a divorce so he could be with this younger woman.

Emotional Experience:

I then asked Françoise, as all her memories resurfaced, to describe the vivid images of her divorce. The scene engraved in her memory was as follows:

After the court ruling, she found herself standing briefly beside Robert at the top of the courthouse steps. Without a word or even a glance, he left her and descended the steps, where his private chauffeur was waiting, holding the car door open. Turning his back on his past, Robert immediately slipped into the luxurious limousine. In contrast, Françoise descended the staircase to the subway entrance, holding her metro ticket in hand, to return to her modest two-room apartment in Paris.

As she descended the steps, she unconsciously recorded her "fall into verticality." She realized she had lost everything: her prestige, her social standing, and her position. The emotional experience of this vertical descent would later manifest as her physical falls years later.

She had fallen down the social ladder, and the image of descending into the metro represented this fall, perfectly in tune with her deep emotional experience.

I proposed that she fully acknowledge this invisible link to neutralize the repetitive cycle around the anniversary of her tragic divorce memory.

Françoise had been stuck in a stage of her grieving process, and this consultation helped her move forward.

Summary:

Understanding allows for a new **A**cceptance. It opens the doors to **H**ealing and enables each of us to break free from the emotional cage and **E**volve on our life path.

Understanding
Acceptance
Heal
Evolve

Françoise never again experienced an accidental fall during that period of the year.

Story No. 5:

SILENCE IS GOLDEN, SPEECH IS SILVER

This is the story of David, the second child in a family of three children (two boys and a girl): Alexandre, David, and Eden, the youngest.

David is a rather introverted child, very attached to his parents, and not inclined to interact with others.

At about four and a half years old, during his second year of kindergarten, his teacher calls his parents to inform them that he is showing, in her opinion, a delay in speech. She insists that it is urgent to schedule an appointment with his pediatrician to establish a medical diagnosis, potentially requiring intervention, and, of course, to keep her informed.

If this speech disorder does not improve, they will need to consider the possibility of placing little David in a special school, as, based on her professional experience, continuing a regular education would only add to his suffering and could permanently hinder his learning abilities.

His parents, shocked by this bad news, immediately make an appointment with Dr. Paul B., an experienced pediatrician who has been passionately practicing for about sixty-five years by 2002.

Consultation No. 1:

The Medical Diagnosis

After a brief inquiry into the reason for the consultation regarding speech delay, Dr. Paul B. proceeds with a thorough examination. With over thirty-five years of experience in private practice, he conducts a palpation examination in front of the astonished parents, explaining the information he gathers through his touch. His findings are as follows:

He explains that David has a short tongue tie, which limits the full movement of the tongue's seventeen muscles. This restriction hinders the tongue's ability to contact the palate, teeth, and cheeks, thereby disrupting the production of sounds that speech therapists refer to as palatal, dental, and labial sounds.

Note: Dr. Paul B. explains that it is unfortunately impossible to surgically cut the tongue tie at this stage. This procedure must be done before the age of nine months, as the floor of the mouth has not yet developed the small artery that would later travel through the tongue tie. This vascularization ensures the blood supply necessary for the tongue's muscular function.

In summary, David suffers from:

• Hypotonia of the diaphragm, which affects the regulation of pressure between the abdominal and thoracic cavities.

• Hypotonia of the abdominal muscles, leading to a decrease in muscle tone.

- Hypotonia of the tongue muscles, causing difficulties with speech (his tongue is described as soft, appearing split in two by a median groove, whereas it should normally be toned).

- Atresia of a vocal cord, causing weakness and fragility in sound production.

All of these clinical findings confirm a real delay in speech development. In conclusion, the machine that produces sounds is broken.

The doctor's treatment is as follows:

- An urgent prescription for speech therapy sessions, one session per week for twelve months.
- Rehabilitation of the tongue muscles by a specialized physical therapist, also one session per week for twelve months.

The parents urgently schedule appointments with these two healthcare professionals.

For an entire year, every Thursday is systematically reserved for appointments, both in the morning and afternoon. David's father takes on the responsibility of attending these sessions, also being allowed to participate in them, as it is crucial to repeat all the exercises at home, in front of a mirror, to optimize progress.

Time is running out, and despite the efforts of the therapists, David, and his parents, no progress is noticeable in correcting this speech delay. Deeply concerned and burdened by this looming fear over their son's future, the parents' stress intensifies. They scour the web, searching for stories of parents facing similar difficulties. During the darkest period of their journey, a glimmer of hope shines through—the discovery of the work of Drs. Claude Sabbah and Gérard Athias.

These two doctors had been giving lectures in France and Europe for the past twenty years on the impact of transgenerational trauma and stress. It is from this point that the parents discover the unexplored world of psychogenealogy.

At the beginning of the lecture, these two doctor-authors speak about the emotional stress experienced by both parents, transmitted and recorded by the fetus during the gestation period. This in utero phase unconsciously influences the psychological, behavioral, and biological future of our descendants. Clara and Jean-Michel, David's parents, agree to make an appointment with a psychotherapist trained in the transgenerational psychogenealogy approach. That is how they end up at my office.

Consultation No. 2:

The Psychogenealogical Approach

This consultation offers the client a way to understand:

- The meaning of the symptom.
- The understanding of the trial.

After carefully listening to David's story, I provide Clara and Jean-Michel with a summary of all the useful information regarding unconscious transgenerational conflicts, in order to resynchronize the memories of their emotions, still bound by invisible ties, inaccessible to their understanding and consciousness.

I then provide the following information to help them grasp the essential principles of this approach.

IMPORTANT CONCEPTS FOR THE READER

Before continuing, it is essential that the reader becomes familiar with some fundamental laws and principles underlying this approach, which has evolved over time through the work of well-known authors (Dr. Claude Sabbah, Dr. Gérard Athias, Anne Ancelin Schützenberger, Jean-Philippe Brebion, Nina Canault, etc.).

The Birth Imprint

This concept originates from the work of Jean-Philippe Brebion. This approach, inspired by the syntheses of several authors and enriched by bio-analogy, seeks to offer a different interpretation of illness. According to Jean-Philippe Brebion, in his book *Twenty-Seven Months for a Life*:

This period spans:

- The nine months preceding our conception.

- The nine months of our gestation.

- The nine months following our birth.

During these twenty-seven months, the embryo records the lived experiences and feelings of its parents. This birth imprint establishes a biological cycle that we will follow throughout our lives.

Guilt

This automatic and unconscious recording of «lived experiences» occurs simultaneously, unbeknownst to both the parents and the embryo. This means that no parent consciously places a burden in their child's cradle, and thus they cannot be held guilty.

There is neither a culprit nor a victim, only the opportunity to recognize the chance life gives us to heal this transgenerational wound or suffering. Only from this moment of realization does our parental responsibility come into play, enabling us to better understand the meaning of illness and of life's trials, elevating our level of awareness and allowing us to transform or even cancel a limiting predisposition. This work is an essential step in our individual, familial, and collective evolution.

Main Laws Related to the Parental Project

- A child unconsciously carries out most of the programs of their parents. Some of these programs can lead to illnesses (illnesses by proxy).

- Illness is the perfect solution to the psychological conflict that the brain of the ancestors cannot manage.

- The brain never makes mistakes; it is programmed to generate the best survival responses within a given context.

- For every illness, there is a "sickening word" and a "healing word"—a word that pushes us into illness and its opposite that brings us back to health. This healing word restores meaning to the patient's survival.

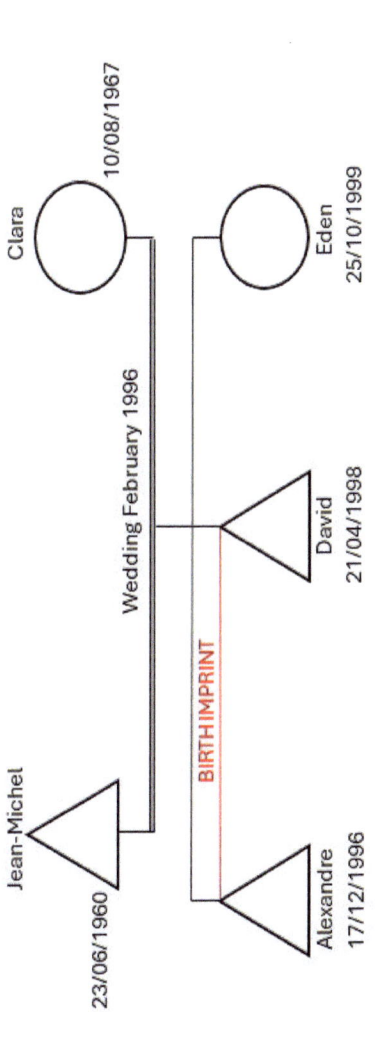
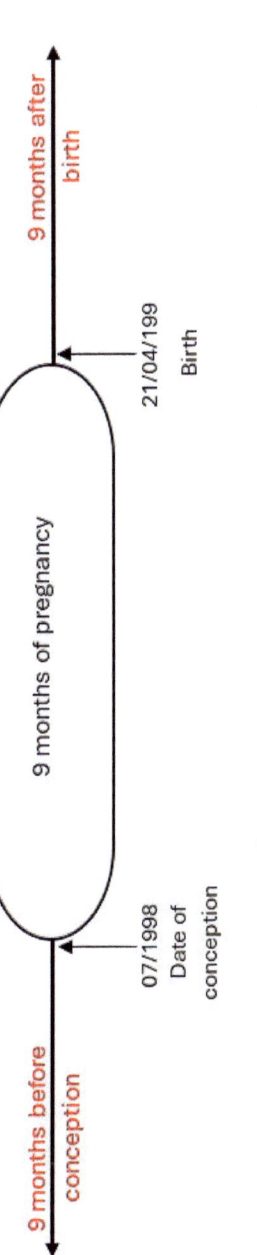

Birth imprint: (Cf.: Jean-Philippe BREBION)

The greatest STRESS PERIOD will last 3 months, from the 3rd to the 6th month of pregnancy, during which David records all the stress from his two parents.

BIRTH IMPRINT ≈ 27 MONTHS

MAIN BIO-PSYCHO-GENEALOGICAL LAWS

- All children are unconsciously «manipulated» by the unmanageable stress of their ancestors.

- Ancestors transmit memories to the family lineage. These memories can be related to stress, specific dates of particular positive or negative events, behaviors, illnesses, or accidents.

CONFLICT EXPERIENCED BY DAVID'S PARENTS DURING PREGNANCY

Story: Retrospective Investigations

- During the second trimester of Clara's pregnancy, David's parents stopped speaking to each other for three months. Communication was almost completely cut off.

- Whenever words were spoken, a violent argument ensued, or a long, painful silence would settle in, with no words exchanged at all.

- David internalized one hundred percent of this stress and was unconsciously tasked with calming the emotional turmoil of his parents, who were unable to resolve their conflict. T

- his biological response manifested in David's speech apparatus, with his tissues encoding a solution: to prevent verbal warfare between his parents.

- To avoid conflict: it was imperative to stay silent. And thus, for David:

"SILENCE IS GOLDEN, SPEECH IS SILVER."

At this point, the meaning of the symptom becomes clear. The previously invisible link is now brought into full consciousness.

Overwhelmed with emotion, Jean-Michel and Clara are devastated by the impact their discord has had on their son's life. A deep sense of guilt arises, along with the immense responsibility to do everything in their power to resolve this issue. Despite the emotional storm accompanying this realization, the parents feel a deep sense of relief, as they finally see a potential solution.

Healing Phase No. 1: Partial Resolution

Protocol:

You must talk to your son, David. Find the right words for a child of four or five years old, and recount your experience in the form of stories or children's tales. Take the time to reflect, reconnect with the emotional tone of the conflict you experienced, and your brain will help you select the words that will «resonate-reason» with your son's feelings.

The parents take time to recall that difficult period in their relationship. Three months pass before the right moment presents itself on a Saturday morning, when David joins his parents in bed while Alexandre and Eden are still sleeping. Jean-Michel and Clara seize the opportunity:

"David, while you were in mom's belly, you knew all the words in the dictionary. You spoke better than Alexandre and Eden. But while you were growing in mom's belly, we fought for three months. Sometimes we wouldn't speak at all, and when we did, we argued loudly. Today, that's all over, but three months is a long time. That's why you still remember those arguments. Now, you see that we talk without yelling or getting angry. At worst, we have small arguments, like you do with your classmates, your brother, or your sister. We argue, then we forget and become friends again. You must forget those fights. You heard the shouting from mom's belly, but today it's over."

David listened quietly for about ten minutes, then simply smiled.

The healing process begins the second the realization occurs. However, fifteen to twenty days are needed for the brain to automatically unfold all the stages of the repair-restoration program. This timeframe is similar to the time required for post-operative healing after surgery, for example.

The moment of realization cancels the biological program associated with the illness: the return to normality happens as the symptoms or behavioral issues gradually disappear. This time frame varies for each individual, depending on their biological rhythm.

Result: Little David recovered eighty-five percent of his speech delay in the two weeks following this realization.

Consultation No. 3:

Consolidation Assessment

A follow-up appointment is scheduled with Dr. Paul B.

- The tongue tie is stretched: length and elasticity are normal.
- The diaphragm: normal tone.
- The abdominal muscles: normal tone.
- The tongue: no more median groove, normal tone.
- The vocal cord: healed.

The remaining fifteen percent of the issue is David's inability to correctly pronounce the letter L.

<u>A follow-up appointment is scheduled with the speech therapist.</u>

She confirms the progress made and assures that David's pronunciation of the letter L will improve with time.

<u>A meeting with the teacher is also arranged.</u>

She, too, acknowledges the remarkable progress in David's speech and behavior in group settings.

The sword of Damocles is no longer hanging over David's head, and the weight on his parents' shoulders has lifted, leaving them relieved and happy with this unexpected resolution.

By mutual agreement, I suggest that the parents take stock in three or four weeks. On the one hand, to assess the progress made by David in pronouncing the letter L. On the other hand, to review their parents' family records in order to construct their family tree over three or four generations, with the aim of elucidating the origin of the pronunciation difficulty with the letter L.

Indeed, the brain never creates a symptom or disorder without "meaning." I therefore explain to them how this information may be stored in the brain using a form of encoding more commonly known as "the language of the birds."

The Language of the Birds: This linguistic approach assigns alternative meanings to words through phonetic play, wordplay, or letter symbolism. This auditory correspondence plays with hidden meanings, anagrams, and subtle coding techniques inspired by the mystical traditions of alchemy and hermetic poetry (from Hermes, the patron of hidden knowledge). It incorporates esoteric figures, syllable or letter permutations, and fragmented words, either to reinforce and amplify the meaning of words or to conceal information.

This language of the birds took on a psychological dimension in the 20th century, notably through the works of Carl Gustav Jung and Jacques Lacan, who identified it as an unconscious encoding mechanism that enhances the meaning of words or ideas.

Consultation No. 4

The Story of Clara's Paternal Family

<u>Objective of the Session:</u> Try to understand the mispronunciation of the letter L.

David's parents attend their follow-up appointment, bringing information gathered from Clara's family. Before reading the family tree, I explain to Clara and Jean-Michel, David's parents, that the unconscious brain spells the letter L in four phonetic forms:

- The letter L.
- The pronoun "she" (elle).
- The verb "hailing" (hèle) in its infinitive form.
- Wing (aile).

These four phonetic possibilities cover the same sound. The question posed to the family—and to which they must find the answer—is as follows:

"WHO IN THE FAMILY LOST THEIR WINGS AND DID NOT GO UP TO HEAVEN?"

It is then that David's parents discover two absolutely unthinkable, unimaginable, and almost inconceivable events for the human mind.

Family Tree No. 2:

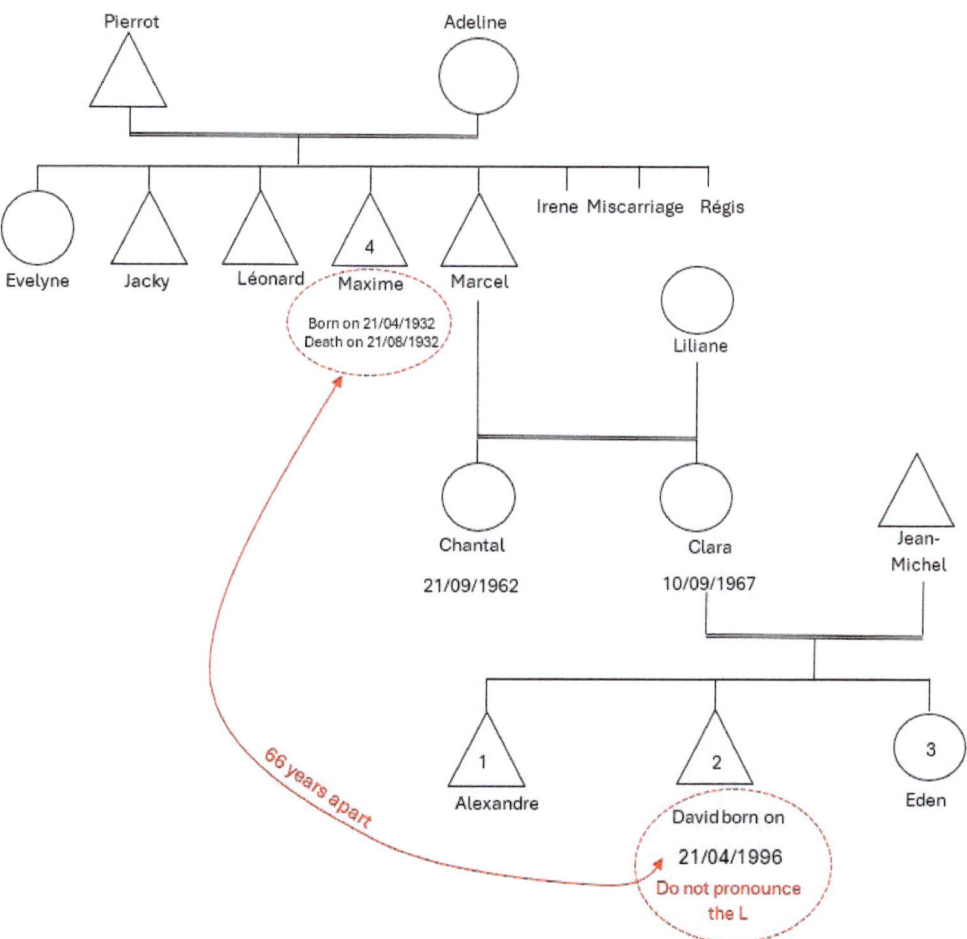

Clara's father, Marcel, is the fifth child in a family of eight children. His mother, Adeline, gave birth to her fourth child, Maxime, on April 21, 1932, who died at four months old on August 21, 1932, from dysentery, which led to his death by dehydration.

The parents, Pierrot and Adeline, devastated by the loss of their child, considered that they had lost an innocent little angel, pure and without sins. They buried their child without performing any religious rituals or eulogies because for them:

"A FOUR-MONTH-OLD BABY IS LIKE AN ANGEL"

AND

"AN ANGEL DOESN'T NEED PRAYERS TO GO UP TO HEAVEN."

Clara and Jean-Michel understand, at that precise moment, that Maxime's soul never symbolically ascended to heaven because the ritual was never performed according to their religious community's customs. Moreover, they discover a previously invisible link: Maxime and little David share the same birth date—April 21, sixty-six years apart to the day.

An incredible coincidence, but a very real one: there is a direct connection between Maxime and David.

This link offers the family the opportunity to proceed with the ritual and allow Maxime's soul to ascend to heaven.

The Ritual Celebration - Protocol

The parents follow my recommendations to carry out the ritual.

- They visit the cemetery with their three children and other close family members, to pilgrimage to the tomb of Adeline, David's great-grandmother.

- Marcel recites prayers in memory of his older brother Maxime for the rest and elevation of his soul.

- Upon returning home, I ask Marcel to take his grandson David on his lap and explain that his great-uncle Maxime has now gone up to heaven, where he rests in peace in a beautiful garden because he finally regained his «L» wings to ascend to heaven.

Results:

After approximately three weeks, little David began to pronounce the letter «L» perfectly.

Observations:

This entire ordeal was orchestrated by the family memory to heal Maxime's soul. These conflicts were imposed on the family by ancestors to contribute to the healing of the family tree. The descendants are tasked with finding solutions to the unspoken secrets and silences of their ancestors.

Each individual's free will evolves and is acquired through consciousness. David's birth date was imposed by his family as a key witness to the realization and repair ritual for Maxime's soul.

NOTE:

Since then, David obtained his baccalaureate in the scientific section with honors, pursued a brilliant academic career, and is currently in his fourth year of aeronautical engineering studies—another story involving wings—as he works toward earning his aeronautical engineering degree.

Story No. 6:

PRIMARY SCHOOL DURING 1939-1945 OR THE VERTIGO OF RUMORS

This is the story of an elderly woman, now 82 years old, who was hospitalized in a psychiatric clinic following chronic depression, worsened by the death of her husband after 58 years of marriage.

I work as a freelance physiotherapist at this establishment, regularly providing care for musculoskeletal issues.

Her two daughters live in the south of France.

During her stay, her psychiatrist prescribed treatment for balance and walking issues, concerned about the risk of a fall. The goal of this preventive rehabilitation was to teach her to stand, walk, and manage stairs safely, maintaining her walking abilities and autonomy for her eventual return home.

At her age, a fall from standing height, especially with potential fractures of the pelvis, lumbar spine, or femoral neck, could have serious consequences, including complications from prolonged bed rest (pressure sores, circulatory problems, phlebitis, muscle atrophy).

I visited her room and, after discussing her medical history, suggested taking a walk through the clinic's hallways to better assess her condition. She agreed. I asked her to hold onto my arm to give her a sense of security.

As we began walking, I noticed several unusual behaviors:

• She immediately lowered her center of gravity by bending her knees and leaning forward.

• With her head down and shoulders hunched, she quickened her pace in an energetic, almost running manner. Her breathing became fast and shallow.

Concerned, I asked her to stop and advised her to take deep breaths. I explained that walking like this could cause the very fall she was trying to avoid.

She responded:

"It's stronger than me, I can't help it. I feel ashamed." She then politely apologized.

I asked her again to hold my arm, follow my pace, close her eyes, and focus on my voice. I repeated her own words back to her:

"You are safe. We are going to ask your unconscious brain to help you remember a time in your life when you felt the uncontrollable need to quicken your pace, felt ashamed, and lost control, with your head down and short, labored breaths. You don't need to make any effort—your brain will take you back in time. If you see an image, hear a sound, or smell something specific, just tell me what your brain has brought back to you: 'Where are you? What are you doing?'"

Note: The NLP technique I used is based on the BioReprogramming® method, a form of conversational hypnosis where the subject is fully conscious but communicates in a state of relaxed focus. This type of communication initiates an emotional recall and helps connect both recent and distant memories. I asked if she could remember this memory while continuing to walk calmly and breathe deeply.

A memory quickly surfaced, her brain connecting in a fraction of a second to a particular episode from her childhood.

The Memory Scene:

She began to recount…

She was with her older sister, who was eight years old. She herself was only six, but the memory remained vivid. It was four o'clock, school had just ended, and, as usual, they had to leave the school and head home.

This small village, with only a handful of inhabitants, was under German occupation. The village had one main street, which they had to cross entirely because the two girls lived with their mother at the far end.

On one side of the street was the school, and on the other was their home. Houses lined the main street, where other schoolchildren lived.

However, a rumor had spread through the village, accusing the girls' mother of having contact with German officers. In that dark period of history, this was a serious accusation.

Every day after school, the girls were heckled and insulted by the other children in the village. To escape the sneers, accusations, and even stones thrown at them, the two sisters would run as fast as they could, heads down, to avoid the projectiles. They would quicken their steps, risking a fall during their frantic escape. The mixture of aggression and shame was something her brain had never forgotten, though it had repressed it for 76 years.

She had been unable to consciously connect her current balance and walking issues to this deeply buried episode from her childhood.

I explained that a significant stressor, like the death of her husband, likely reawakened certain traumatic episodes from her life.

By becoming aware of the invisible link between this painful childhood memory and her current symptoms, our conversation gave her the opportunity to understand, accept, and heal.

She was finally able to let go of the shame and dishonor that had been imposed on her family.

Her balance and walking issues gradually improved in the days following this realization, and eventually disappeared entirely.

At the end of her hospitalization, she returned to her Paris home.

The brain never forgets, and the body never lies.

Story No. 7:

SANTA CLAUS OR THE CHRISTMAS TREE IN THE CLINIC

This is the story of a 39-year-old woman named Christelle, who works as a medical secretary in a psychiatric clinic. I worked there regularly as an osteopath-physiotherapist, treating musculoskeletal issues for patients with depression, personality disorders, mood swings, phobias, and paranoia.

It was winter 2008, and the world outside was cloaked in an immaculate white blanket of snow. The trees were burdened with heavy layers of snow, and the branches drooped under the weight. Occasionally, a gust of wind would shake the snow free, and it would fall to the ground with a muffled thud, while the liberated branches seemed to spring upwards, reaching for the sky.

The clinic was nestled in a verdant park with century-old trees, one of which was a magnificent red spruce standing proudly at the entrance. Its monumental branches spiraled up to the sky like a staircase. The morning sun cast a golden light across the electric blue sky.

At 8 a.m., I parked my car in the clinic's staff lot and noticed Christelle standing near the elevators, sneezing repeatedly. Her eyes were red and watery, and she apologized, explaining that she hated the Christmas season. Each year, she developed an allergic reaction affecting her nasal, sinus, and eye mucous membranes. Her entire ENT (Ear-Nose-Throat) system was affected, despite treatment from her allergist. She had already undergone all desensitization tests and discovered she was allergic to pine trees, spruces, and specifically the molds found in these trees, which are potent seasonal allergens.

Her allergy manifested as:

- Eye irritation,
- Runny or stuffy nose,
- Cough,
- Fatigue.

I asked her when these symptoms first appeared.

Christelle replied, "Only five years ago. Before that, I never had any allergies. As for why it started, I have no idea—it's just a seasonal allergy."

Investigation - Retrospective:

If her body had developed these symptoms, which persisted despite treatment, it was likely in response to an unresolved, emotionally painful situation. This seasonal allergy pointed us to a specific time: the end-of-year holiday season, celebrated between December 23 and 31. The fact that it had started five years ago also gave us a clue about the onset of the symptoms.

I asked Christelle to listen calmly to the sound of my voice and let her brain recall a moment, a sequence.

"What was happening in your life between Christmas and New Year's in 2003?" I asked.

At that moment, her automatic brain recalled a painful scene where her entire life had changed in an instant. She recounted:

"I remember it clearly. We were all gathered at my parents' house, happy to have the family together—my parents, my sister, our husbands, and all the grandchildren. The traditional meal was served, and all the gifts were placed under the Christmas tree by the fireplace. Everyone was excited, young and old. Then, suddenly, my sister and my husband stood up and announced, 'We've been living a double life for two years, and we can't lie to ourselves or the family anymore. We're in love and are leaving tonight to be together!"

They left, walking out on the entire family, leaving us stunned by the sudden and brutal announcement. I was shocked and humiliated. My husband was leaving me for my sister! My parents were in disbelief; none of us had suspected anything. It felt like the world collapsed in a matter of moments.»

After this cataclysm, divorce proceedings began, and the grieving process was set in motion.

Synthesis:

I asked Christelle if she could now recognize the connection between her "Christmas tree allergy" and the deep emotional pain from the betrayal she experienced during Christmas 2003. I explained that to protect her from the overwhelming emotional hurt, her brain had activated a survival mechanism: avoiding contact with the allergen (the Christmas tree) as a way to shield her from that moral suffering. The Christmas tree had become the emotional symbol of that family tragedy.

In that moment, Christelle understood that her allergy was a biological response triggered by her brain. This new understanding, coupled with her acceptance, allowed her to enter the healing phase and begin to overcome the allergy.

For years, Christelle had worked at the clinic and expressed her allergy to Christmas tree molds only between December 23 and 31 each year. Yet for the rest of the year, she walked past the same magnificent red spruce every morning without any symptoms. Her brain, much like a computer, recorded the rhythms of time and space, and this spatio-temporal reactivation occurred only on the anniversary of the event, when her emotional and unconscious stress peaked.

Since then, Christelle has rebuilt her life, sharing her days with a new partner, who also has two children. She realized that she couldn't change the past or control others, nor could she alter the external world. By viewing her life story through a different lens, she fostered a new emotional understanding deep within herself. This inner peace alleviated her moral pain, gradually allowing her to reconnect with her sister and ex-husband.

Forgiveness became a crucial step in healing her emotional wounds, enabling her to achieve physical recovery.

Today, all symptoms of her allergy have completely vanished, and Christelle no longer dreads Christmas family celebrations!

Story No. 8:

ECZEMA ON BOTH HANDS OR THE FATHER'S DEPARTURE

This is the story of a 55-year-old man, Laurent B., living in the Paris region.

Laurent has been married for about 20 years and is the father of three children. He works as a financial advisor in an analytical firm.

In April 2016, Laurent consulted me for the first time due to dysfunction in his temporomandibular joint, primarily affecting the right side.

This condition is known as SADAM (Syndrome Algo-Dysfonctionnel de l'Articulation Mandibulaire) or Costen's Syndrome.

Definition and Symptoms:

This widespread condition causes pain and a variety of symptoms, including:

- Jaw popping and limited movement,
- Tinnitus (ringing or buzzing in the ears),
- Temporal and ear pain,
- Headaches,
- Dizziness,
- Neck pain,
- Fatigue.

Treatment typically involves physiotherapy and/or osteopathy to relieve muscular and ligament tension and often requires a psychotherapeutic approach.

During the sessions, Laurent revealed that he also suffered from chronic eczema on both hands for several years, despite treatments from his general practitioner, dermatologist, and allergist.

The condition flared up sporadically, alternating with periods of remission, without a clear understanding of the triggers. Various prescriptions provided temporary relief but failed to eradicate the recurring episodes.

I then suggested exploring the possibility of a psycho-emotional approach as a complementary treatment to conventional methods.

Consultation No. 1:

Reason for Consultation: Eczema on both hands.

Definition: Chronic inflammation of the skin that flares up episodically. It is a form of dermatitis that alternates through four stages:

- Erythematous phase,
- Vesicular phase,
- Weeping phase,
- Crust phase.

These stages coexist in various forms, but itching and pruritus are constant. Healing occurs without scarring, followed by the next cycle of recurrence.

Eczema on the hands can be particularly debilitating, affecting daily life and progressively lowering quality of life, often leading to work absences, sleep disturbances, depression, and social phobias.

The goal of treatment is to achieve an "inactive" eczema state, improving psychosocial well-being.

To help Laurent understand the psycho-emotional approach, I briefly explained the key principles of this method.

KEY CONCEPTS:

The External World

Humans are constantly in contact with the external world throughout life, even from the womb, where a fetus can already hear the voices of its parents and the sounds of its environment.

This communication with the external world happens primarily through our five senses, which filter the reality around us:

- Hearing: sound, music, voices (the ears),
- Sight: images, light, colors, (the eyes),
- Taste: flavors, food, spices (the tongue),
- Smell: aromas, perfumes, scents (the nose),

- Touch: contact, temperature, separation (the skin).

All of this happens in a dynamic interplay with space, movement, and time. Humans are connected to the world through a spatio-temporal dimension of their environment, although selective memory may distort experiences, creating emotional conflicts that manifest as symptoms, diseases, or behavioral disorders.

The Brain: A Super-Computer

Our brain records our life history, storing all events and experiences. Its primary function is to keep us alive, adapting moment by moment to a sometimes hostile environment. It regulates all the body's vital functions and organs, controlling the processes of repair, healing, and homeostasis.

The brain launches repair processes when the individual becomes aware of their emotional conflicts, most of which are experienced in isolation and without coping strategies. The resulting emotional upheaval can manifest as physical symptoms, diseases, or behavioral issues.

Understanding the Symptom:

Questions:

- Why eczema?
- Why is the disease localized on the hands?
- How can we understand the recurrence cycle?
- How does this disease reflect Laurent's emotional experience?

The Session:

I invited Laurent to undergo a sensitivity test commonly used by neurologists to assess fine sensory disturbances. This test involves distinguishing between two stimuli, such as a prick and a touch, performed on different areas of the body.

I asked Laurent to close his eyes and tell me whether he felt a prick or a touch, and whether he sensed contact or separation. He had to locate the exact point of contact on his hands:

- Finger (palmar, dorsal, lateral, or pulp),
- Phalanges, nails,
- Thumb, index, middle, ring, little finger,
- Palm or back of the hand,
- Right or left side.

This test highlighted that the skin is the organ of touch, containing millions of receptors that record fine sensory details. At the end of the test, I explained that skin diseases are often related to the pain of separation. The skin tries to communicate an emotional story of **»contact and separation.«**

A person may experience:

- Loss of contact (with a family member, friend, or pet), associated with regret and sadness, a pure separation,

- Imposed contact (with work, a superior, or a partner), where separation is desired but delayed.

Laurent realized that we would need to investigate a painful separation, either from a lost contact or from an imposed relationship he longed to escape. We scheduled another session 10 days later.

Consultation No. 2:

LOCATION: BOTH PALMS.

Laurent asked why the eczema was located specifically on his hands.

EXPLANATION:

In the collective unconscious, humans are seen as a bridge between Heaven and Earth.

This concept is fundamental in Traditional Chinese Medicine (TCM), where humans are understood in relation to their external environment, connected to both Heaven and Earth: hands reaching toward Heaven, feet firmly rooted in the Earth.

- Yang: the masculine principle linked to Heaven,
- Yin: the feminine principle linked to Earth, the nurturing mother.

The hands are symbolically, emotionally, and unconsciously linked to Heaven (the Father), while the feet are linked to Earth (the Mother).

At this moment, Laurent made the connection and told me his story.

April 18, 2013:

Laurent received a phone call informing him that his father had been admitted to the emergency room. Though he was reassured that his father's condition was stable, the news was concerning.

Laurent's father was 79 years old and had been receiving treatment for several years for:

- Kidney failure, possibly requiring dialysis,

- Insulin-dependent diabetes for about 30 years,

- Heart failure, which had required triple coronary bypass surgery in 2007.

Despite the excellent care provided, Laurent's father passed away on May 13, 2013, in Paris. He was buried the next day, May 14, in Ashdod, Israel.

Laurent and his brothers, from a traditional Jewish family, recited daily prayers for the elevation and rest of their father's soul, following the tradition for the first year of mourning and then annually on the anniversary of the death.

Laurent's eczema was an expression of the deep pain associated with his father's death. I explained that in all monotheistic traditions, prayers are offered with palms turned toward Heaven, as if to receive the divine offering.

Laurent was deeply moved. His emotions overwhelmed him, and he wept as he recounted the following memory:

THE MEMORY SCENE:

"We were at the synagogue for Rosh Hashanah, the Jewish New Year, in October 2016. I was overcome with sobs I couldn't control. As always, we were gathered under my father's prayer shawl (talith). His children and grandchildren stood together as my father recited the annual blessing, placing his palms on each of our heads. In that moment, I felt the profound absence—those two protective palms would never again rest on my head during the New Year's blessing."

LIBERATION AND SYNTHESIS:

Laurent understood intellectually and emotionally the unconscious link between his eczema and his father's death.

The skin represents separation, and eczema was the expression of this painful emotional separation. The palms of his hands symbolized the connection to his father and to Heaven. Accepting this helped release the stages of his grief.

CHANGING THE PERSPECTIVE:

I suggested that Laurent now consider blessing his own children during the New Year, just as his father had done, passing the tradition from one generation to the next. This realization allowed Laurent to finally find peace with the emotional pain of separation, understanding that his father, from above, was asking him to carry on the tradition.

CONCLUSION:

A few weeks later, Laurent's eczema had completely healed, without scarring, and there has been no recurrence since 2016.

This realization allowed his brain to release the body from the emotional burden, restoring biological balance and homeostasis.

NB: REMINDERS TO THE READER

THE TALITH: Definition

In Jewish tradition, it is a prayer shawl, worn by individuals while praying. This concept emphasizes the idea that we are all equal before the Creator. The shawl is typically made of wool or silk, adorned with fringes at its four corners, called tzitzit. The talith is worn during morning prayers. The wearing of the talith is a commandment that symbolizes the entirety of the commandments, reminding us of our obligation to fulfill the six hundred and thirteen laws stated in the Torah.

Eczema Photos 2013-2016

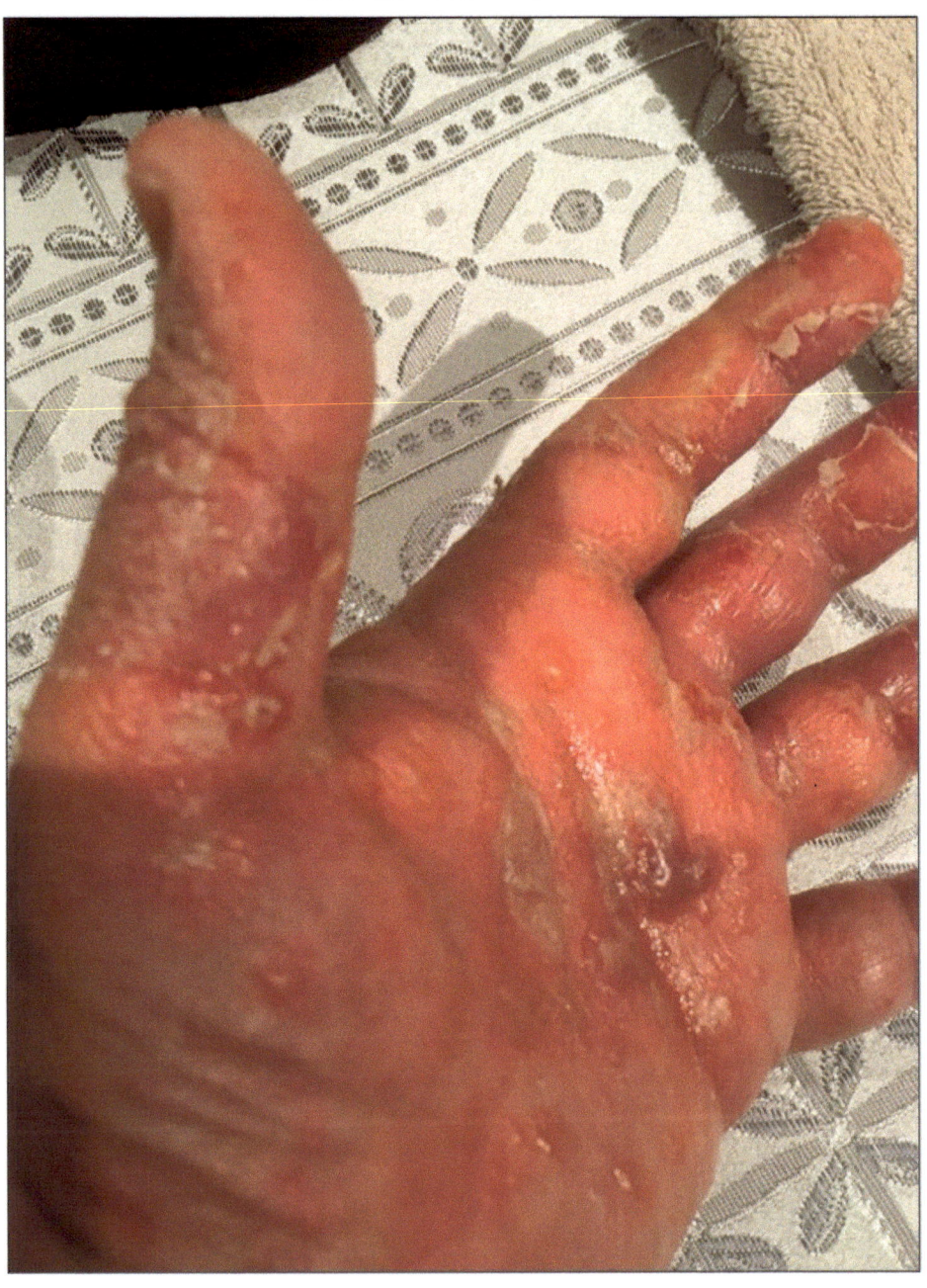

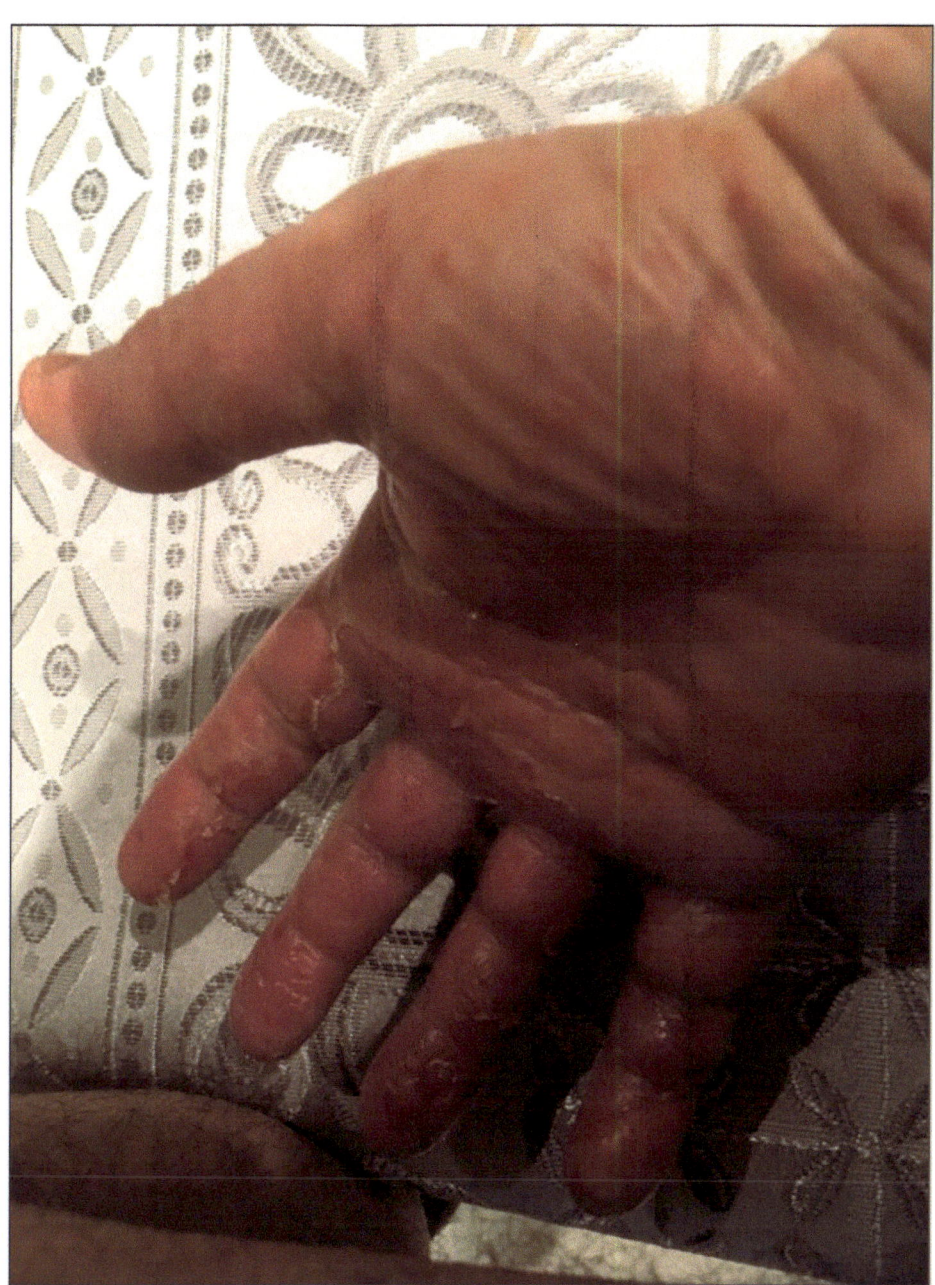

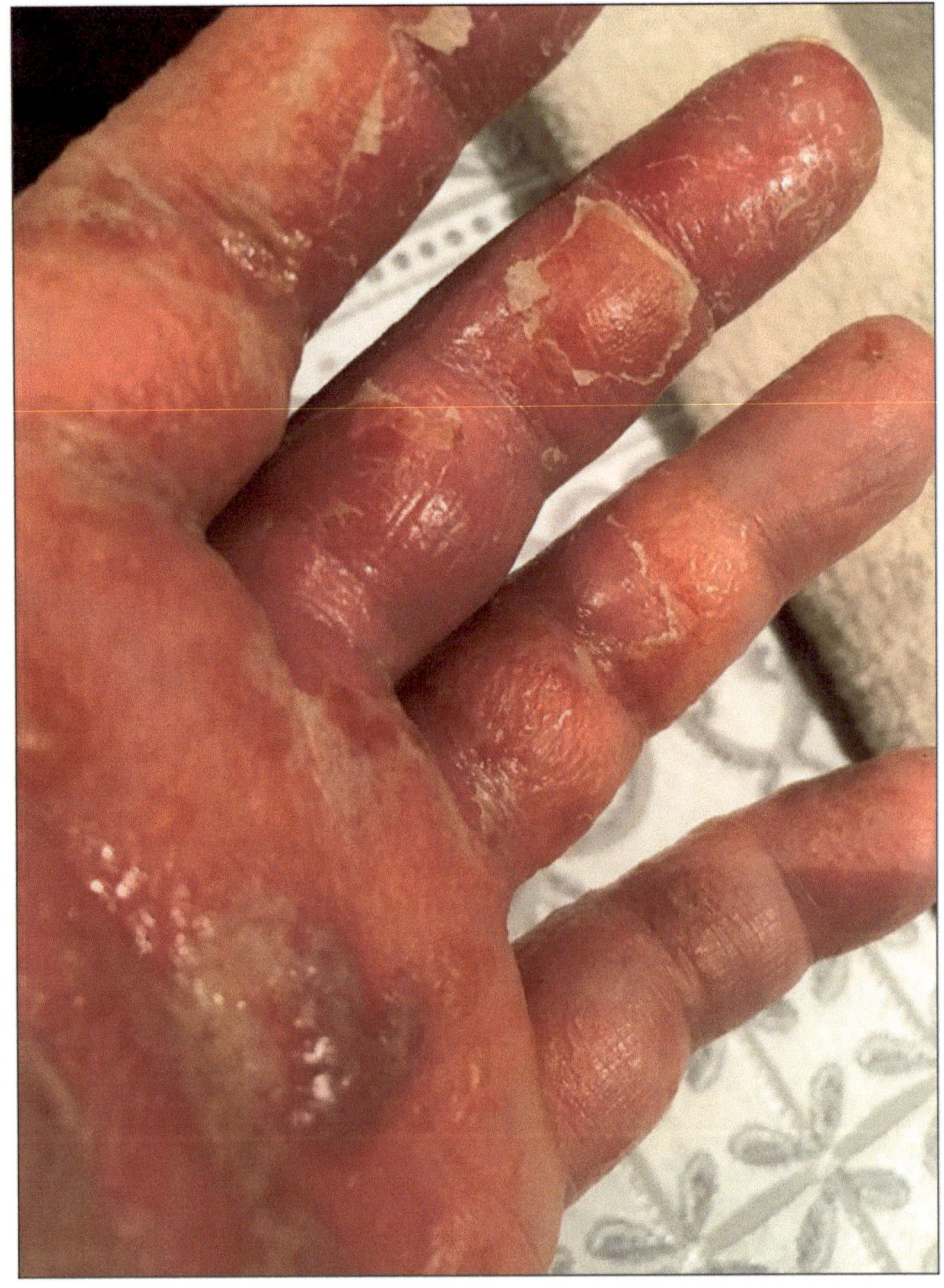

Photos 2016-2023: Healing

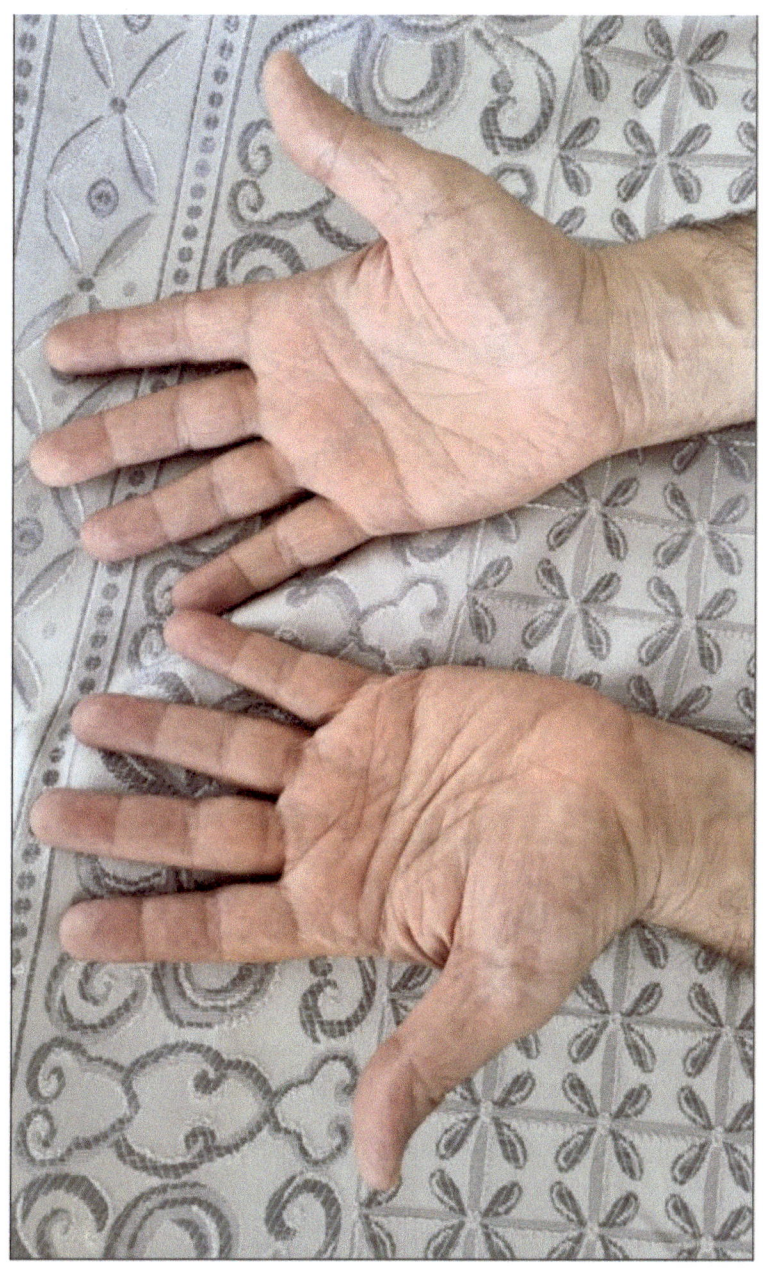

Story No. 9:

THE LAST METRO OR IT'S ONLY A GOODBYE

Hélène is a 67-year-old woman who lives in the Paris suburbs, in a small town in Val-de-Marne (94). She used to work as a commercial manager for members in a large Parisian mutual insurance group, and she has been retired for about ten years.

Her reason for consulting: "insomnia resistant to any treatment."

INSOMNIA[3]

Definition: Insomnia affects approximately one in five people in France (20% of the population). Its frequency increases with age and is considered severe in 9% of cases. It affects the quantity and/or quality of sleep and includes the following symptoms:

- Difficulty falling asleep,
- Nighttime awakenings,
- Early morning awakening without being able to go back to sleep.

[3] Source INSTITUT NATIONAL DU SOMMEIL ET DE LA VIGILANCE

Fatigue quickly affects mood quality, disrupting work efficiency. Recovery phases, or even falling asleep, cause concentration and attention issues, and the socio-professional impact is constant.

Occasional or transient insomnia is often related to lifestyle and environmental disturbances (noise, light, excessive heat or cold, defective bedding, stress, anxiety, illness, disregard for healthy living habits). Once the cause is identified and removed, insomnia ceases immediately, and normal sleep is quickly restored.

Chronic insomnia, however, occurs at least three times a week for more than three months. It then requires the investigation of pathologies such as hyperthyroidism, gastroesophageal reflux, asthma, depression, inflammatory rheumatism, sleep apnea, and restless legs syndrome.

Consultation No. 1

Questioning

Hélène confirms that she has undergone all the assessments and complementary examinations successively prescribed by her general practitioner and various specialists (neurologist, pulmonologist, cardiologist, ENT) to find a cause for her stubborn insomnia. All her tests came back negative.

The prescribed treatments:

• Anxiolytics, antidepressants, mood stabilizers, hypnotics,

• Melatonin-based treatments, the so-called sleep hormone, which does not regulate sleep rhythms.

All these remedies provide temporary relief but are too short-lived to offer significant recovery. She then confides, as if to justify her approach:

"Anyone who suffers, no matter how resilient, is always eager to find a lasting solution to their illness or symptom. Over the years, I naturally turned to other therapeutic options such as acupuncture, homeopathy, reflexology, massages with essential oils selected for their calming and relaxing properties, and shiatsu, a traditional Chinese massage performed according to the meridians of acupuncture. I must admit that none of these therapies brought significant relief."

Thus, she came to my practice after discovering on some internet forums that cranial osteopathy could offer an answer to her issue.

OSTEOPATHIC ASSESSMENT

I proceed with a palpatory assessment in osteopathy, while asking her to confirm if she has experienced a recent or even very old trauma (from a fall from standing height, or resulting from a direct impact, a public road accident, etc.):

- On the top of the head (the vertex),
- On the cervical vertebrae,
- On the lumbar spine, pelvis, coccyx, sacrum.

Hélène does not recall any recent or old traumatic incident.

I continue my palpatory investigation:

- Palpation reveals nothing objective that could substantiate a relevant link between our patient's insomnia and craniosacral tension.
- Furthermore, the tissues at the base of the skull and cervical tensions release easily with osteopathic maneuvers: no mechanical barriers resist the manipulative techniques.

NOTE: CRANIOSACRAL THERAPY

In osteopathy, traumas transmitted to the fascia, aponeuroses, and soft tissues can create tensions affecting the meninges (pia mater, arachnoid, dura mater). These three fibro-hydro-connective membranes protect the entire central nervous system, extending from the skull to the base of the spine: the sacrum and coccyx. Inside the skull, the dura mater extends into two folds: the falx cerebri and the tentorium cerebelli. Thus, there is a physical continuity between the skull, its contents, and the base of the spine. This anatomical reality underlines the concept of «craniosacral» therapy in osteopathy. The release of these reciprocal membrane tensions facilitates the rebalancing of the craniosacral axis, which can lead to various symptoms, including insomnia, migraines, vertigo, headaches, and tinnitus.

Consultation No. 2

The second appointment, scheduled eight days later, showed no improvement following the previous session. The clinical picture remains absolutely identical: there is no change.

Objective of this consultation: to understand the meaning of the symptom.

I then explain to Hélène that the persistence of symptoms, combined with the absence of objective biomechanical tension, may open the way to a different but complementary interpretation. At this point, I mention a psycho-emotional approach, as stressful emotions are stored and remembered in our body's cells.

This feeling, tied to a psychological episode experienced dramatically, imprints itself deep within our tissues: our cellular memory. Most of the time, this automatic recording occurs unconsciously, without our knowledge. Our brain uses this automated process to prevent the patient from experiencing unbearable emotional suffering daily. The brain's goal is to eventually convert this emotional shock into a physical symptom, but only if it cannot develop a conscious solution or defense strategy. This is how illness or behavioral disorders arise, as the brain functions like a fuse box. An organ and/or its function are used, or even sacrificed, preserving the rest of the body, which continues to ensure the individual's survival. This program is our brain's best biological response. This solution resonates perfectly with the emotional conflict and tone of the situation. This response is not random but perfectly orchestrated, and it is essential to understand that continuous stress systematically puts any individual at risk, gradually depleting their energy reserves, which can lead to death from exhaustion and/or lack of vigilance. Although the price is illness, the patient remains alive for a certain time, giving them the opportunity to find a satisfactory solution. It is precisely this time that should be used to attempt to reverse, consciously, the morbid process.

Hélène accepts this approach. I then invite her to lie down on the osteopathy table, comfortably positioned on her back, with both arms extended along her body, resting on the armrests.

I place my hands on her skull, as if for an osteopathic session, and simply ask her to listen, feeling safe, to the sound of my voice:

"You can, if you wish, close your eyes. We are going to ask your automatic and unconscious brain to travel back in time and help us understand why it was useful for you to develop this symptom or illness: this insomnia resistant to all treatment, despite the care provided by the medical field. This new interpretation suggests analyzing your insomnia as the best biological response your brain devised, echoing a stress or an unmanageable situation at a precise moment in your life."

Here is the continuation of the story translation:

EXPLANATIONS TO THE READER

It is necessary to allow the patient to reconnect with the emotional experience linked to the onset of their symptom, while respecting a spatial-temporal framework.

I use a communication method similar to conversational hypnosis. This Neuro-Linguistic Programming (NLP) technique employs a sophronic relaxation method. This slightly altered state of consciousness allows the patient to connect to their recent or old memory. The induction aims to activate the parasympathetic system, thereby stimulating a state of relaxation, deep and full breathing, and an inward focus in the patient.

PHYSIOLOGICAL REMINDERS

It is important to specify that the autonomic nervous system is composed of two essential components for the survival of living beings: they are complementary, relative, and in constant interaction.

- A stimulating system, called the sympathetic system, which is essential for fighting, acting, and defending the individual in case of alert, combat, or flight. It is active during all our dynamic activities, movements, and displacements. It is located mainly along the spine and represents the paravertebral ganglionic chain. This system is regulated by two neurotransmitters: adrenaline and noradrenaline.

- A braking system, called the parasympathetic system, or the vagus system, is active during periods of rest, repair, and relaxation phases. It induces a general slowdown in the organism's functions. The vagus nerve, or the 10th pair of cranial nerves, represents the largest part of this system, mainly located in the cranial and pelvic areas. This vagus system promotes sleep, dream activity, sexual relations, and appetite stimulation. It is associated with a neurotransmitter: acetylcholine.

In this type of approach, the hypnotic induction, created through speech, is associated with touch by the therapist's hands placed on the cranial vault. This double action (auditory and tactile) encourages the stimulation of the parasympathetic system, and the patient-therapist dialogue can begin.

Session:

"Hélène, how does it feel to live with this, this daily insomnia?»

"It's unbearable and it exhausts me.»

"What do you feel?»

"I can't do anything about it; it's just how it is. There's no solution despite all my efforts. It's been almost nine years.»

I rephrase her feelings carefully, using the words Hélène herself has spoken:

"Hélène, for the past nine years, you've been facing an exhausting and unbearable situation without being able to change anything, despite all your efforts. You don't have to do anything specific, just allow yourself to be lulled by the sound of my voice, as we ask your automatic and unconscious brain to travel back in time and space, to when you faced an exhausting, unbearable situation.»

A few seconds pass as her brain switches into automatic search mode, replaying scenes imprinted in resonance with her feelings. Her brain reconstructs and selects a sequence of evocative memories.

<u>MEMORY SCENE:</u> She begins to recount

"Yes, nine years ago, I was going to visit my mother in the evening to have dinner with her during one of her hospital stays in a Paris service. She was being monitored and treated in the terminal phase of breast cancer, with respiratory and pulmonary complications. I made it a point to be there every day. You understand, I am her only child, and since I have no children of my own, I felt it was important, after work, to be there for her and share her day and her evening meal. I had been with her during each of her successive hospitalizations and, of course, I had the opportunity to get to know the different medical teams. Very devoted staff, understanding, and always listening, they even allowed me to stay late in the ward. One evening, a nurse came to tell me I should go home because my mother was very tired and needed rest and quiet. She reassured me, saying that I could leave with peace of mind and that if anything happened, they would call me immediately. According to her, nothing significant would happen until the next day. That night, I left the hospital around 11 p.m., hurried to catch the last metro, and got home around midnight. After a quick wash, I went to bed and fell asleep around 1 a.m. I was abruptly awakened at 5 a.m. by the phone ringing. On the other end of the line, the night nurse was telling me that my mother had passed away peacefully in her sleep."

As I listen attentively to all the details of this memory scene, I understand that all the elements related to her insomnia are present in her story. However, it is impossible for Hélène to discover and understand this connection consciously.

It is now up to me to reassemble the thread that will allow Hélène to grasp the hidden meaning, while also uncovering the emotional aspect of her insomnia. This conscious understanding enables acceptance, releasing the body, which has become both the prisoner and guardian of her symptom. Hélène is stuck in one of the various stages of grief and cannot move towards healing. Indeed, understanding the deep meaning of her illness allows her to accept it, paving the way to the program of restoration-repair and leading her on the path to healing.

EXPLANATIONS:

Hélène continues to listen to the sound of my voice, her eyes closed, my hands still resting on her cranial vault.

"Hélène, could you please specify the time at which your sleep disturbances occur?"

"I am unable to sleep between 1 a.m. and 5 a.m."

SYNTHESIS: I OFFER HER ANOTHER INTERPRETATION OF HER INSOMNIA

"Hélène, your brain has chosen the best possible strategy to cope with your stress, perfectly reflecting your situation regarding your mother's death. This response is your optimal biological reaction at that moment in your life. Each evening during the week, when you leave your mother, your emotional stress heightens as you silently fear not being present when she takes her last breath. You cherish every minute spent with her. Thanks to the understanding and empathy of the medical teams, you postpone the moment of separation each night, which hints at an inevitable and permanent parting. During your last visit, you left the hospital quite late, and your mother was still alive at that time. After returning home, washing up, and closing your eyes, exhausted from those consecutive days, it was around 1 a.m. At that moment, your mother was still alive. However, at 5 a.m., you were suddenly awakened with the news you had been dreading: your mother had passed away. It is precisely this time frame that your brain selected: from 1 a.m. to 5 a.m.

- 1 a.m. = life,
- 5 a.m. = death.

For your brain, as long as you don't sleep, your mother is still alive. The insomnia keeps you awake, symbolically keeping your mother alive: 'As long as I'm awake and not asleep yet, my mother is still alive,' or 'That night, as soon as I close my eyes, my mother leaves me.' This unconscious emotional phrase has been etched into your brain, feeding your cellular memory: this insomnia unconsciously soothes your stress related to your mother's death. You must prolong the wakefulness phase and avoid sleep, hence the insomnia between 1 a.m. and 5 a.m."

At that moment, Hélène understands and consciously accepts this invisible connection. She finally realizes the burden of guilt she has been carrying for nine years: she has never accepted her absence, and she deeply regrets, from the bottom of her soul, not being present that night.

LETTING GO:

Hélène refuses to forgive herself for her absence, for leaving, for sleeping that night. This self-accusation prevents her from going through the different stages of grief.

RECONTEXTUALIZING THE FACTS:

Hélène is still lying on the osteopathy table, eyes closed, listening to the sound of my voice. My hands remain on the base of her skull. I must now try to change her perception. I explain to her that no one on Earth has the power to change events. They belong to the past; we can only change or evolve our feelings, looking at things from a different perspective.

"Hélène, the loved one who leaves us often, or almost always, chooses the moment when they are alone so as not to impose on those they love, on their relatives, the face of death, the last breath, the death rattle of their final exhalation, doing this so that the memory of life remains engraved in their loved ones' minds."

While continuing to listen to the sound of my voice, Hélène has relived the entire scene of that last night with great emotion. Tears stream down her face. I encourage her to hold on to and relive the moment when she said goodbye to her mother.

"Being present and watching 100% of the time is impossible. To set oneself this mission is unattainable. The most important thing is to consider all the support and love you offered through your tender care and presence, not just those few moments your mother chose for her departure."

Hélène has accepted to reconsider the framework and limitations of her presence at her mother's bedside. She has accepted to let her mother go. She has finally been able to complete her grieving process.

Consultation No. 3

We scheduled a third appointment fifteen days later, allowing her brain time to resynchronize the biological rhythms of her sleep.

Since then, Hélène has been sleeping like a baby again, feeling serene about her care and support for her mother. She is at peace with herself once more.

EXPLANATION AND SYNTHESIS

Note to the reader: The constant progress of medicine and the power of pharmaceuticals allow the boundaries of disease to be pushed back while optimizing the preservation of health. However, it is sometimes essential to understand that any chronic symptom or illness recurrence may require a complementary approach to medical care.

INDEED:

- **THE BODY NEVER DEVELOPS OR MAINTAINS A SYMPTOM WITHOUT MEANING.**
- **THE BODY IS THE GUARDIAN OF THE MEMORY OF OUR SOUL'S WOUNDS.**
- **THE BODY NEVER LIES.**
- **AS LONG AS EMOTIONAL SUFFERING IS ACTIVE, THE BODY EXPRESSES THE SYMPTOM.**
- **BECOMING AWARE OF THE LINK BETWEEN EMOTIONAL SHOCK AND THE SYMPTOM CANCELS THE DISEASE PROGRAM, ALLOWING THE BODY TO ACTIVATE ITS HEALING PROPERTIES.**
- **THIS AWARENESS ALLOWS THE RELEASE AND COMPLETION OF THE DIFFERENT STAGES OF GRIEF.**

Story No. 10:

RIB FRACTURES OR THE VIOLENCE OF THE FATHER

Brigitte comes to my osteopathy practice due to recurrent back pain. She is about forty years old. She is clearly a stylish, well-groomed woman: elegant figure, large almond-shaped green eyes, a few freckles highlighting her prominent cheekbones, a high forehead, a proud gait, and an abundance of black hair cascading down to her lower back. All of this gives her a beautiful presence.

REASON FOR CONSULTATION: BACK PAIN

I ask her to specify the circumstances in which her spinal pain appeared. She replies without hesitation that it occurred following rib fractures about ten weeks ago. In the event of any trauma, a radiological assessment must be done on the day of the accident, followed by a check-up within three or four weeks to monitor the healing process. I ask her to show me the X-rays to review the report from her radiologist.

Indeed, any delay in the healing process is a contraindication for osteopathy sessions. She has come without any additional tests or X-rays. I then ask her to clarify the circumstances of her rib fractures to assess whether the intensity of the trauma corresponds with a general weakness or other issue.

Did the problem occur due to:

- Traumatic shock: fall from standing height, sneezing, stress fractures?
- Metabolic disorders: demineralization, osteoporosis, nutritional deficiencies?
- Hormonal disorders: thyroid, adrenal glands, parathyroid glands?

Irritated by my questioning, she asserts that she is fine and wants me to quickly relieve her spinal tensions, which she believes are the result of her fractures. I explain to her that I cannot perform osteopathic manipulation without knowing the context of her fractures, as they may indicate a deeper issue with her overall health. I ask her to return with the radiological exams and to schedule another appointment.

"It's safer for you," I tell her.

She then asks me what I want to know, as, according to her, her general practitioner didn't ask so many questions. This statement leaves me perplexed, as I cannot imagine that her family doctor would overlook these details. For reasons I don't understand, I sense she doesn't want to provide more explanations.

"I prefer to respect, without compromising, the fundamental principles related to the practice of osteopathy and postpone this appointment until you bring your exams and radiology reports.

These precautions are taken with your best interest and medical safety in mind."

"Alright, she finally admits. «I just ask that you don't reveal the content of our discussion to my general practitioner, as we've reported this accident to occupational health. Do you understand?"

"Rest assured, I just want to understand the context of your fractures. I don't represent nor work for any social service or regulatory agency. This conversation remains strictly confidential."

"We had a violent argument, my husband and I, which happens quite often. He pushed me to the ground, and I landed hard on my left side, then he delivered a violent kick to my right side, causing the rib fractures on both sides. There, now you know everything. Believe me, the radiological check confirmed the fractures were healing. That's why my family doctor allowed me to return to work four days ago."

"Brigitte, thank you for your testimony and your trust. If your doctor approved your return to work, that reassures me regarding the healing of your rib fractures. Brigitte, before proceeding with the session, do you have any other medical history I should be aware of?"

Brigitte doesn't understand the meaning of my question and immediately responds:

"Yes, this is the third time!"

As if the history of frequent arguments should have made it obvious that her husband had, logically, broken her ribs for the third time.

"Brigitte, I fear I didn't hear or understand your answer correctly. Did you say this is the third time your husband has broken your ribs?"

"Sorry, you misunderstood. It's not just my husband: three times, by three different men."

Indeed, I no longer understand anything about this conversation. I'm literally stunned by Brigitte's revelations, as she seems to accept this without much emotion about the recurring nature of the situation. Although her story seems completely surreal to me, I pause, a look of astonishment undoubtedly crossing my face. A few seconds pass, but they feel like an eternity. In my mind, I can't help but say aloud, though only to myself, this phrase that still resonates like a silent echo:

"Is ALL of this even possible, let alone acceptable, without raising the slightest question? Could this be a dark joke about her own life, a way to heal herself from her own tragedy?"

Doubt begins to creep in. Although completely destabilized by her story, I return to the consultation, which now seems more like a scene from a science fiction movie or a nightmare from another world.

"Brigitte, before continuing, allow me to express my complete confusion about the course of your story. If you'd like, we can take a few moments to try to understand why and how you are experiencing such a repetition in the script of your life. I know life isn't always logical; some events are hard to grasp. However, for your well-being, it's sometimes necessary to try to understand the meaning and content, if you are, of course, willing."

"What are you trying to make me understand? I don't get the point of your questioning, your surprise? What answers are you referring to? This is my life; that's how it is, and I'm forced to accept it. I can't do anything about it; I just live with it. You know, I deeply loved those two men in the past and still love the one I'm with today."

EXPLANATIONS:

I offer Brigitte another approach, another way to understand.

"I don't doubt for a second the strong and genuine bonds you shared with these three partners. What puzzles me in your story is this seemingly inevitable repetition. I must explain that I work, in addition to musculoskeletal trauma, on emotional and unconscious wounds that can trigger recurring, repetitive life events. These daily life challenges can be driven by unconscious programs. They act without your knowledge, like magnets, forcing you to attract the same types of people or situations to continue this inexplicable repetition, defying all the laws of chance and statistics. To put it simply: if you constantly experience the same injuries, it's because you are subject to these repetitions, even if they escape your conscious awareness. Your honesty and sincerity are not in question; simply accept the possibility of being helped to understand the hidden and still invisible meaning to your emotional consciousness."

"I've never considered the situation in these terms. I'm sincere, you can believe me. But I'm willing to try to understand."

"Brigitte, just answer these few questions. (Without giving her further explanation, I seek to understand the nature of her relationship with her masculine archetype.)

Who is the most important man in the life of a woman, a wife?"

"Her husband."

"Very well, and for a little girl?"

"Her father."

She immediately adds, laughing as if to ward off what's coming next:

"That has nothing to do with this. My father has been dead for a long time."

"Brigitte, excuse my question, but what did your father die of, if you don't mind?"

"Alcoholism, alcohol poisoning."

At the mention of her father's death, she continues spontaneously, her memories flooding back, and emotions punctuate her speech. Her pace slows, her voice becomes quieter. A silence follows, and then she resumes:

"With my two brothers and my little sister, when we heard the sound of car tires crunching the gravel in the driveway, we would all run and hide in the house. We feared his fits of anger and, often, violence. Our mother was always the first target of this violence, which she couldn't control or stop. Then it was the children's turn to suffer his outbursts, his blows. Drunk with anger and alcohol, he would collapse in the hallway, passed out. This misery was our childhood. We lived in constant fear of the next outburst."

"Brigitte, how old were you when your father died? Where were you at that precise moment?"

"I was eight years old and still in school. When we returned home with my brothers and little sister, our mother gave us the sad news."

Brigitte cries uncontrollably, finally admitting to me:

"You know, my father never held me or took me in his arms. I never received a single gesture of affection from him. It's terrible. I have no memory of ever being in his arms, and most of all, I never said goodbye to him."

The passage of time since her father's death hasn't diminished the intensity of her memories. The images etched in her memory are very vivid. Between sobs, she repeats that recalling that period of her life remains deeply painful. Overwhelmed, she cries for several minutes.

QUESTIONS – ANSWERS

Without her understanding the invisible connections that weave her life story, her testimony contains all the details of this sad repetition. I pose the following questions to her:

"Brigitte,

- Why and how have three different men in your life subjected you to the same grim scenario? Understand that this repetition defies all laws of chance and statistics.

- Why have three physical assaults by three different people occurred in the same place on your body: your fractured rib cage on both the right and left sides?

- What macabre staging are you the victim or target of?

"I don't know; I'm unable to answer you."

"You regret not being able to say goodbye to your father. This feeling is legitimate, but it contributes to blocking the different stages of your grieving process. You can ask your adult self, the woman you are today, to bring resources by addressing the wounded little girl still within you. What could you say or advise this eight-year-old girl to do?"

I then ask Brigitte to close her eyes and reconnect with that difficult moment, imagining herself as the younger version of herself.

"I can advise this child to imagine that her father, from wherever he is, is tenderly holding her in his arms. I can also advise her to go to the cemetery to say goodbye to him."

"Brigitte, thank you for offering these resources to your younger self, because your unconscious emotional brain has been reliving, on loop, the only connection you still had to your father. Your response was, unknowingly, to choose violent men to continue maintaining this emotional bond with your father: as long as your father is violent, he is alive. To keep your father symbolically and unconsciously alive, you refused to acknowledge the moment of his death, blocking the various stages of grief. These stages—sadness, anger, guilt, incomprehension, and finally acceptance—could not unfold. Your unconscious mind kept making you experience this violence on repeat."

At that moment, Brigitte begins to understand the endless cycle of these life episodes. She consciously agrees to break free from this invisible link. Before letting her leave, I suggest that she visualize one last time the image of her father tenderly embracing her, wrapping his arms around her rib cage, to feel and experience that embrace. This step is essential to finally dissolve the relationship that was based on violence, allowing a space for love and tenderness to take its place.

EPILOGUE

We scheduled another appointment about fifteen days later to release the tensions related to the aftermath of these fractures. After the session, Brigitte thanked me for my work, for the time I had given her, and for helping her.

"You've helped me understand that I've always attracted violent men into my life to relive and re-experience my relationship with my father. By the way, I must confess that I've never felt anger or bitterness towards the men in my life. I've just now realized why. I sincerely thank you for that."

I never saw her again in my osteopathy practice. I sincerely hope that her life has been lightened of this burden so she can live and build a new relationship with the masculine.

Epilogue:

FROM ORIGINS TO THE PRESENT... FROM TODAY TO TOMORROW.

Since the dawn of time, faced with an often hostile external world, humans have continuously adapted to ensure the survival of the human species.

In response to the increasing dangers, ingenious survival systems have been developed. Thanks to the evolution of the human brain, solutions have been created to ensure the transmission of life, under all circumstances and conditions. Nowadays, the brain is compared to a supercomputer where each illness corresponds to a mathematical solution.

This response is a perfectly memorized and orchestrated program, rooted in the patient's archaic emotions. This emotional coloring is an authentic representation, containing the smallest details of what the patient has felt and experienced. It is this feeling that embeds itself deeply into our cells, potentially causing a disruption.

Each spatio-temporal stress results in a logical response from the body in the form of an illness or behavioral disorder within a specific context.

For each of us, this response resonates in perfect harmony with our mental world, emotions, life experiences, inner filters, and transgenerational memory.

Thus, this approach seeks to utilize the rapid advancements in neuroscience, which have provided numerous insights toward a revolutionary understanding of illness. This new, broad-spectrum perspective offers patients the possibility of stimulating and connecting multiple areas of their brain.

In this way, an original path opens up for a more varied and expansive understanding of the links between the expression of a pathology and our personal history.

I hope that this humble presentation can offer the greatest number of people the opportunity to consciously participate in the stages of their own healing.

A process is evolving, as an invitation to a deeper and more intimate inquiry into our inner selves. Each of us can share the fruit of this new knowledge with the rest of humanity.

An infinite gratitude to all the actors of this extraordinary journey. See you soon for new adventures on the path to Healing.

BIBLIOGRAPHY

Les racines familiales de la maladie, tomes 1-2-3, Dr Gerard ATHIAS, Éditions PICTORUS

Le corps point par point, Dr Gerard ATHIAS, Éditions PICTORUS

Questions-Réponses avec Gerard ATHIAS, Forum Internet 2005, Éditions PICTORUS

Biologie Totale Des Êtres Vivants, tomes 1-2-3-4, Dr Claude SABBAH, Auto-éditeur

Dictionnaire Des Codes Biologiques Des Maladies, Dr Eduard Van Den BOGAERT, Éditions TELIGATE-ASBL

La Psycho généalogie expliquée à tous, Mme Anne Ancelin SCHUTZENBERGER, Éditions PAYOT

Aïe, mes aïeux !, Mme Anne Ancelin SCHUTZENBERGER, Éditions PAYOT

Exercices pratiques de psycho-généalogie, Mme Anne Ancelin SCHUTZENBERGER, Éditions PAYOT

L'Empreinte de Naissance, M. Jean-Philippe BREBION, Éditions QUINTESSENCE

Comment paye-t-on les fautes de ses ancêtres, Nina CANAULT, Éditions DESCLEE DE BROUWER

Comprendre, accepter... Guérir, Dr Philippe DRANSART, Éditions LE MERCURE DAUPHINOIS

La Psycho généalogie Appliquée, Paola Del Castillo, Éditions QUINTESSENCE

La médecine sens dessus dessous, Giorgio MAMBRETTI et Jean SERAPHIN, Éditions AMRITA

La Médecine Nouvelle « La Quintessence », Dr Ryke Geerd HAMER, Éditions AMICI DI DIRK -ESPANA

Origine Des Cancers, Dr Michel MOIROT, Éditions LES LETTRES LIBRES

Et si LES MALADIES étaient des MÉMOIRES DE L'ÉVOLUTION, Dr Robert GUINEE, Éditions NEOSANTE

POUVOIR ILLIMITÉ, Anthony ROBBINS, Éditions GODEFROY

The BIO-BREAKTHROUGH, Mᵉ ISABELLE BENAROUS, Bio reprogramming Press LOS ANGELES CALIFORNIA

Atlas des techniques manipulatives des os du crâne et de la face, Alain GEHIN, Éditions MAISONNEUVE 1981.

Biomécanique et pathologies crâniennes en étiopathie, Michel Altiéri, Éditions Etiosciences SA, Geneve 1984.

Vision toucher relation thérapeutique, René LAVATELLI-Étiopathe D.E Auteur-Editeur, Édition 1999.

ACKNOWLEDGEMENTS

To my wife, Sophie

My most loyal support since the beginning of this journey... With all my love and tenderness.

To my children

By trying to answer all your questions, you unintentionally nurtured and deepened in me the need to write.

I love you,

BERNARD

To my lifelong friend,

For your unwavering support, your generosity, enthusiasm, availability, our camaraderie, and your friendship...

For introducing me one day to osteopathy... and bio-psycho-genealogy...

THANK YOU

I thank all the professors at the European College of Osteopathy in Geneva for the quality of their teaching and their availability...

A special thought goes to Mr. Jean-François TERRAMORSI, Director of Studies, a teacher, and a passionate man.

May he rest in peace.

With all my gratitude and deep respect.

<u>To everyone else,</u>

To the teachers, therapists, lecturers, doctors, psychotherapists, psychiatrists, psychomotor therapists, occupational therapists, sports coaches, art therapists, nurses, healthcare managers, clinic directors, secretaries... may they all be thanked here for their trust, open-mindedness, and attentive listening to me. I have learned so much from their kindness and our exchanges.

<u>To my family</u>

To my grandparents, Michel, Charles, Emma, and Esther

To my father, Jacques, that singing nightingale

To my brothers, Fabrice, Philippe, Emmanuel, and Steve

To their wives, my nieces and nephews

To my mother, Renée, who dedicated her entire life to her five sons…

and her career to the world of children as a childcare assistant within an association responsible for welcoming children born under "X." To heal these birth wounds, armed only with her maternal instinct and remarkable intuition, she would continually address these newborns, simply telling them that life would fill them with love. She would then send her most loyal lieutenant, Jacques, to urgently fetch a disposable camera from the nearest store. She took a concrete step to imprint the memory of these emerging lives: she created for each one a photo album, like an open-hearted book. After a few months, these children found their adoptive families, each entrusted with preserving this precious book of images as a treasure.

Upon discovering their first moments of life, many children, accompanied by their parents, would return years later to revisit this home where they had been fed their first bottles filled with love.

The magical testimony of these children, incredible yet absolutely authentic, is that the memory of this place was imprinted in their cellular memory—without the slightest doubt for them.

Mom pursued two professions during her working life:

• As a seamstress, she wove fabrics, dresses, and trousers. She mended torn clothes until about the age of fifty.

• She practiced her art as a childcare assistant until her seventy-fifth spring. Her mission was to weave connections to mend the torn fragments of a life so that the miracle of rebirth could occur.

Her parents named her well: Re-née, or reborn, to be reborn into life.

THANK YOU FOR THIS GIFT...

A SPECIAL THOUGHT,

To the masters who trained me in this approach, I would like to thank two professionals who contributed to radically transforming my journey of understanding and approaching illness.

First, Dr. Claude SABBAH, an international lecturer for his concept "The Total Biology of Living Beings," described as natural histories of the three kingdoms: plant, animal, and human. This immense work of scientific analysis and synthesis reveals archetypes of survival functioning, offering everyone the possibility of understanding them to better manage their health.

Too often imitated, rarely equaled by those who have used his work, forgetting to pay tribute to this legacy.

CLAUDE, THANK YOU FOR THIS GIFT...

REST IN PEACE...

Infinite recognition to Dr. Gérard ATHIAS for his intuitive intelligence and his ability to make the understanding and interpretation of diseases accessible to many. His constant invitation to explore the heart of genealogical transmissions allows us to discover this genius logic. His unique and so original decoding of our emotions transports us to a world he offers us to discover and explore... from symbol to healing, with the disease expressing an intimate message of our personal and family history.

GÉRARD, THANK YOU INFINITELY...

TO ISABELLE BENAROUS

I appreciate your generosity, insightful advice, unwavering support, and encouragement. Thank you for your detailed feedback, patience, and attentive listening. I am grateful for the exceptional tools you've developed to help people resolve emotional conflicts and for your contributions and passion for this work.

Thanks to you, this project for the first edition can see the light of day.

WITH ALL MY FRIENDSHIP...

Table des matières

ABOUT THE AUTHOR	5
DISCLAIMER TO THE READER	7
INTRODUCTION	9
Story No. 1: **WATER ALLERGY OR THE MEMORY OF A FAMILY TRAGEDY**	13
Story No. 2: **OBSESSIVE-COMPULSIVE DISORDER: KNOCK KNOCK, WHO'S THERE?**	19
Story No. 3: **VAGINAL YEAST INFECTION OR THE ODYSSEY OF LIFE**	25
Story No. 4: **THE SOCIAL ELEVATOR OR THE FALL INTO VERTICALITY**	35
Story No. 5: **SILENCE IS GOLDEN, SPEECH IS SILVER**	39
Story No. 6: **PRIMARY SCHOOL DURING 1939-1945 OR THE VERTIGO OF RUMORS**	55
Story No. 7: **SANTA CLAUS OR THE CHRISTMAS TREE IN THE CLINIC**	59
Story No. 8: **ECZEMA ON BOTH HANDS OR THE FATHER'S DEPARTURE**	63
Story No. 9: **THE LAST METRO OR IT'S ONLY A GOODBYE**	77
Story No. 10: **RIB FRACTURES OR THE VIOLENCE OF THE FATHER**	89
Epilogue: **FROM ORIGINS TO THE PRESENT… FROM TODAY TO TOMORROW.**	99
BIBLIOGRAPHY	101
ACKNOWLEDGEMENTS	103

© Michel-Charles SULTAN, 2025

Translation: ChatGPT with corrections of Sarah UZAN and Isabelle BENAROUS

Layout and cover: Ton livre comme unique

Edition : BoD · Books on Demand, 31 avenue Saint-Rémy, 57600 Forbach, bod@bod.fr

Printing : Libri Plureos GmbH, Friedensallee 273, 22763 Hamburg (Allemagne)

Legal deposit : avril 2025

ISBN : 978-2-3225-5400-3

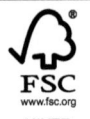